A Competency-Based Framework
for Health Education Specialists - 2020

Copyright ©2020
Second Printing
National Commission for Health Education Credentialing, Inc.
& Society for Public Health Education, Inc.

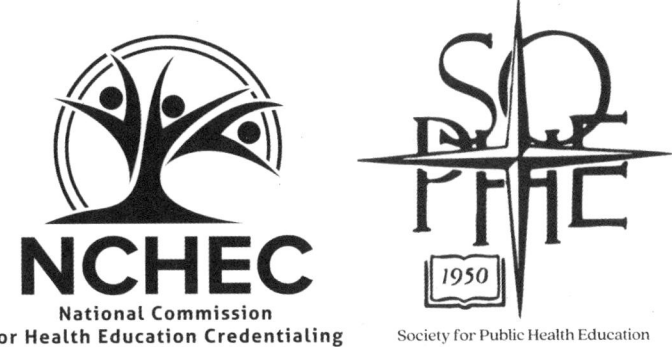

NCHEC
National Commission
for Health Education Credentialing

Society for Public Health Education

A Competency-Based Framework for Health Education Specialists - 2020

For reprint permission or ordering information contact:
The National Commission for Health Education Credentialing, Inc.
1541 Alta Drive, Suite 303, Whitehall, PA 18052-5642
www.nchec.org
888-624-3248

Suggested Citation:
National Commission for Health Education Credentialing, Inc.
& Society for Public Health Education, Inc. (2020).
A Competency-based Framework for Health Education Specialists - 2020.

A

Health Education Specialist Practice Analysis II 2020 Contributors

A qualified, competent health workforce is essential to improving the public's health. The health education profession has contributed to this goal since the 1970s by undertaking multiple, rigorous scientific efforts to identify Competencies that reflect the knowledge and skills needed by health education specialists in all practice settings. This National Health Education Specialist Practice Analysis II 2020 (HESPA II 2020) Model represents the latest evolution of Health Education Competencies, which underlie the profession's commitment to excellence in health education teaching, research, and practice.

The National Commission for Health Education Credentialing, Inc. (NCHEC) and the Society for Public Health Education, Inc. (SOPHE) are proud to lead the health education profession in sponsoring the HESPA II 2020 research and disseminating this publication. SOPHE and NCHEC are the joint copyright holders of this publication and the research data.

An initiative of this breadth and depth would not be possible without the expertise and dedication of many individuals. First, we are deeply indebted to Randall R. Cottrell, DEd, MCHES® and Adam P. Knowlden, MBA, PhD, CHES®, who, as chair and vice-chair of the HESPA II 2020 Technical Advisory Group (TAG), devoted hundreds of hours to guiding

the research conceptualization, implementation, data analysis, and interpretation. Their extensive knowledge of the health education profession, research skills, leadership, and perseverance helped move the project forward in a scientifically rigorous and timely fashion. Second, sincere thanks are extended to James Henderson, PhD of Scantron Assessment Solutions, who was contracted to assist with the HESPA II 2020 project. We are indebted to Dr. Henderson and his staff for their expertise in psychometric research and their overall guidance in professional competency research design, implementation, and analysis. James McKenzie, PhD, MPH, MCHES®, co-chair of the Health Education Specialist Practice Analysis I 2015 (HESPA I 2015) study and Kathleen Allison, PhD, MPH, MCHES®, former SOPHE Trustee and chair of the NCHEC Division Board for Certified Health Education Specialists (DBCHES), also provided invaluable guidance as researchers and members of the HESPA II 2020 TAG. Cynthia Kusorgbor-Narh, MPH, MCHES® spearheaded communications, outreach, and meeting coordination. NCHEC and SOPHE staff are acknowledged for their invaluable support in all phases of this effort.

Finally, our gratitude extends to the Health Education Practice Panel (see Appendix C) and many other volunteers who served in various roles related to study procedures and/or the development of this publication. We thank the

Health Education Specialist Practice Analysis II 2020 Contributors
(continued)

thousands of health education specialists who voluntarily completed the HESPA II 2020 survey, as well as the many professional volunteers who contributed to this publication.

All those who assisted in HESPA II 2020 can take pride in helping pave the way for a health education workforce that is knowledgeable and skilled, and sets our profession apart from other public health and allied health disciplines. We thank you for your contributions and your dedication to promoting and protecting the nation's health.

Elaine Auld

M. Elaine Auld, MPH, MCHES®
Chief Executive Officer, SOPHE

Linda Lysoby

Linda Lysoby, MS, MCHES®, CAE
Executive Director, NCHEC

Contributors to A Competency-Based Framework for Health Education Specialists II 2020

Editor
Randall R. Cottrell, DEd, MCHES®

Contributing Authors
Adam P. Knowlden, MBA, PhD, CHES®
James McKenzie, PhD, MPH, MCHES®
Kathleen Allison, PhD, MPH, MCHES®
M. Elaine Auld, MPH, MCHES®
Linda Lysoby, MS, MCHES®, CAE
David Birch, PhD, MCHES®
Kadi Bliss, PhD, MCHES®
Bridget Cross, MA, CHES®
Chandra Jennings, PhD, MS, MCHES®
Cynthia Karlsson, MPH, MS, CHES®
Cynthia Kusorgbor-Narh, MPH, MCHES®
Suzanne Lineberry, MPH, MCHES®
Elisa Beth McNeill, PhD, CHES®
Kerry Redican, PhD, CHES®
Cherylee Sherry, MPH, MCHES®
Michael Staufacker, MA, MCHES®
Jila Tanha, MPH, CHES®
Jennifer Torres, MPH, CHES®

Reviewers
M. Elaine Auld, MPH, MCHES®
Linda Lysoby, MS, MCHES®, CAE
James Henderson, PhD
Melissa Opp, MPH, MCHES®
Laura Rasar King, EdD, MPH, MCHES®
Cynthia Kusorgbor-Narh, MPH, MCHES®

Copy Editor
Dianne L. Kerr, PhD, MCHES®

A Competency-Based Framework for Health Education Specialists – 2020

Table of Contents

Table of Contents

Table of Contents

List of Tables

List of Figures

A Competency-Based Framework for Health Education Specialists – 2020

The purpose of this publication is to communicate the 2020 Responsibilities, Competencies, and Sub-competencies that are essential to contemporary health education/promotion practice. This document contains descriptions of the processes, outcomes, and related materials of the Health Education Specialist Practice Analysis II 2020 (HESPA II 2020), which replaces the Health Education Specialist Practice Analysis I 2015 (HESPA I 2015). This updated model is designed for use by those in the health education/promotion profession to guide professional preparation, credentialing, and professional development. In accordance with best practices in credentialing excellence, the National Commission for Health Education Credentialing (NCHEC) and Society for Public Health Education (SOPHE) undertake a psychometric study of health education specialists job responsibilities and knowledge every five years and communicate the results to preservice programs and in-service providers to promote excellence in health education.

Section I of this document contains a brief overview of historical perspectives related to the growth and evolution of the health education/promotion profession and its quality assurance efforts. In Section II, the processes and outcomes of HESPA II 2020 are described. In Section III, the resulting HESPA II 2020 Model containing the updated Areas of Responsibility, Competencies, and Sub-competencies for health education specialists is presented. Section IV contains recommended uses of the HESPA II 2020 Model for various stakeholders and 12 specific recommendations for the profession, endorsed by SOPHE and NCHEC leadership, as well as the Coalition of National Health Education Organizations (CNHEO). Section V provides a comparison of the HESPA II 2020 Model with the previous HESPA I 2015 Model. Section VI includes a set of Knowledge items verified in the HESPA II 2020 analysis. The appendices include additional materials that can be used to master professional terminology and adapt professional preparation and development efforts to the HESPA II 2020 model.

We hope this Framework publication will be useful in your efforts to implement the HESPA II 2020 Model in your teaching, research and practice and contribute to our ongoing collective commitment to health education excellence.

The HESPA II 2020 Model continues the ongoing strong commitment of NCHEC and SOPHE to promote excellence in health education research, teaching and practice, as predicated on a psychometrically validated study of health education specialists across all practice settings. The historical perspectives below serve as evidence of this pioneering spirit. This section contains an overview of the first role delineation project and its impact on professional preparation programs and certification; the development of graduate-level Areas of Responsibility, Competencies, and Sub-competencies; the development of the Competencies Update Project (CUP) Model, which led to three levels of practice defined by years of experience and educational degree; and the use of best practice job analysis methods that led to the development of the Health Educator Job Analysis 2010 (HEJA 2010) and Health Education Specialist Practice Analysis (HESPA I 2015) Models. This section also contains information about a series of accreditation task forces that laid the foundation for high-quality professional preparation and practice standards in health education/promotion and strategic directions for program accreditation and individual credentialing.

Role Delineation

The history of health education in the United States dates to the late 19th century with the establishment of the first academic programs preparing school health educators (Allegrante et al., 2004) and later public health educators (IOM, 2003). In the 1940s, interest in quality assurance and the development of standards for professional preparation of health educators began to emerge. Over the next several decades, professional associations produced guidelines for preparing community health educators and introduced accreditation efforts (SOPHE, 1977). Yet, it

was not until the 1970s that health education began evolving as a true profession (Livingood & Auld, 2001). In addition to defining a body of research, SOPHE and other health education professional organizations began to promulgate a Health Education Code of Ethics, as well as agree upon the use of terminology, a skill-based set of Competencies, rigorous systems for quality assurance, and a health education credentialing system.

Long-standing questions about the practice of health educators eventually led to the first Role Delineation Project in the 1970s. In February 1978, health educators from all practice settings assembled at the First Bethesda Conference to begin the process of defining and verifying their role. The stated purposes of the conference were: (a) to analyze the commonalities and differences that existed in the preparation of health educators within different practice settings and (b) to determine the potential for developing acceptable guidelines for professional preparation that would include all practice settings (NCHEC, 1985). The conference attendees recommended the establishment of the National Task Force on the Preparation and Practice of Health Educators, and this recommendation was realized in March 1978. In collaboration with the National Center for Health Education, this task force undertook the landmark Role Delineation Project (United States Department of Health, Education, and Welfare, 1978).

Following considerable public discussion and background research, the Role Delineation Project resulted in discerning the role of entry-level health educators during the years 1978 to 1981. After conducting a national survey of practicing health educators, which helped verify and define the role of the health educator, the leaders of that project concluded that there was a "generic role" common to all health educators. That is, commonalities in the roles and functions of entry-level health educators existed regardless of whether they were employed in schools, communities, health care facilities, worksites, or other settings. This finding formed the basis for health education credentialing and the refinement of academic programs in the United States.

Professional Preparation and Certification

Between 1981 and 1985, the National Task Force on the Preparation and Practice of Health Educators developed a curriculum framework using the defined role delineation research findings. This framework was based on contributions from academics and practitioners involved in two national conferences, several regional workshops, and many meetings of professional associations. The resulting document, *A Framework for the Development of Competency-Based Curricula for Entry-Level Health Educators* (NCHEC, 1985), provided individuals associated with professional preparation programs a standard reference for developing or refining a health education curriculum. A Competency was defined as the "ability to apply a certain specified skill in dealing with some defined amount of meaningful subject matter" (NCHEC, 1985, p. 2). As such, the Framework included Competencies as a reflection of both content and process.

During the Second Bethesda Conference in 1986, attendees reached a consensus that a certification process was appropriate to ensure that individuals delivering health education services possessed a minimal level of competence. Preliminary steps for developing a national certification system for health educators were initiated, culminating with the establishment of the National Commission for Health Education Credentialing, Inc. (NCHEC) in 1988. Following a charter certification phase in 1989, during which individuals who met eligibility requirements could become certified through a review of documentation submitted (e.g., letters of support, academic records), NCHEC offered the first national Competency- based certification examination in 1990. Thus, the

results of the Second Bethesda Conference formed the basis for a: (a) framework for professional preparation, (b) national examination, leading to credentialing eligible individuals as Certified Health Education Specialists (CHES), and (c) guide for continuing education for practitioners (NCHEC, 1996).

Graduate-Level Areas of Responsibility, Competencies, and Sub-competencies

In 1992, the American Association for Health Education (AAHE) and the Society for Public Health Education (SOPHE) initiated efforts to determine graduate-level Areas of Responsibility, Competencies, and Sub-competencies when they commissioned the Joint Committee for Graduate Standards (SOPHE & AAHE 1997). The committee sought the input of individuals involved in graduate-level professional preparation through a national survey and at various annual professional associations' meetings, as well as its own continuing deliberations, to ascertain the advanced-level of practice by health educators with advanced training and experience. The committee projected that its work would build on the entry-level skills within the Seven Areas of Responsibility already identified, as well as establish new Areas of Responsibility at the advanced-level.

Following the publication of a final report and its acceptance by the boards of AAHE, NCHEC, and SOPHE, the Graduate Competencies Implementation Committee was formed. Committee members addressed the ways in which the new advanced-level Areas of Responsibility, Competencies, and Sub-competencies would be disseminated to and implemented by the health education profession. The resulting document, *A Competency-Based Framework for Graduate-Level Health Educators*, was jointly published by NCHEC, AAHE and SOPHE in 1999. This publication also contained a history of the work of the Committee (NCHEC, AAHE & SOPHE, 1999). The results ultimately were re-examined within the National Health Educator Competencies Update Project (CUP).

Competencies Update Project (CUP)

During the mid-to-late 1990s, approximately a decade after the first role delineation project, professional organizations and individual health educators felt there was a need to re-verify the role of entry-level health educators. To accomplish this, NCHEC initiated the National Health Educator Competencies Update Project (CUP) in 1998, a study with the participation of AAHE, SOPHE, and nine other national health education related organizations. This multiphase national research study was guided by the CUP National Advisory Committee, consisting of representatives of the 12 national professional groups and a three-person CUP Steering Committee (Drs. Gary Gilmore, Larry Olsen and Alyson Taub) that led the project with assistance from research expert Dr. Dave Connell (Gilmore, et al., 2005). The project included a planning and resource development phase (1998-1999), a survey development and pilot process phase (2000-2001), and a four-year data collection, analysis, and reporting phase (2001-2004).

An updated model from the CUP study included Seven Areas of Responsibility, 35 Competencies, and 163 Sub-competencies (Gilmore et al., 2005). Based on statistical analyses and professional judgment, the CUP Hierarchical Model emerged with implications for professional preparation, credentialing, and professional development. The CUP Hierarchical Model identified three levels of practice, each building on the other, defined by years of experience and degrees:

- **Entry-level**: less than five years of experience with a baccalaureate or master's degree

- **Advanced 1-level**: five or more years of experience with a baccalaureate or master's degree

- **Advanced 2-level**: five or more years of experience with a doctoral degree

A new edition of *A Competency-Based Framework for Health Educators - 2006* (NCHEC, SOPHE, & AAHE, 2006) was published based on the CUP results.

During the same time frame as the CUP study was undertaken, SOPHE and AAHE convened the National Task Force on Quality Assurance in Health Education to examine issues related to quality assurance in professional preparation and practice of community and school health educators (Allegrante, et al., 2004). Following multiple meetings (including NCHEC leadership) and several surveys, the task force issued a report in 2003 with recommendations to the profession to eliminate confusion and to provide a vision for strengthening quality assurance of the health education profession.

Based on the SOPHE/AAHE National Task Force on Quality Assurance in Health Education's recommendations and the CUP results, SOPHE, AAHE, and NCHEC issued four recommendations that were unanimously endorsed in 2006 by the Coalition of National Health Education Organizations (CNHEO). These recommendations included preparing students in baccalaureate and graduate programs to perform all Seven Areas of Responsibility, with baccalaureate students expected to demonstrate proficiency at the entry-level, and graduate students expected to demonstrate proficiency at the entry- and advanced-level Competencies and Sub-competencies of the CUP Model. In addition, it was recommended that NCHEC base the entry-level certification examination on entry-level components of the CUP Model (Airhihenbuwa et al., 2005).

HEALTH EDUCATOR JOB ANALYSIS 2010 (HEJA 2010)

To keep pace with societal and population health issues, and to meet the accreditation standards of the National Commission for Certifying Agencies (NCCA) (see the "Accreditation of the CHES® and MCHES® Certification Programs" section of this publication for more information on accreditation of credentials), the Health Educator Job Analysis (HEJA 2010) study was launched in 2008 and completed in 2009. For the first time, an independent agency, Professional Examination Service (ProExam), was contracted to assist with the reverification process to ensure best practice in workforce competency development and analysis in a timely manner. To complete the project, ProExam experts partnered with a five-member steering committee (i.e., chief staff officers of NCHEC, SOPHE, and AAHE, the 2008 coordinator of the NCHEC Division Board for Certification of Health Education Specialists, and the appointed HEJA 2010 task force chair (Dr. Eva Doyle), an 11-member task force, and 49 volunteer subject matter experts, independent reviewers, and survey pilot participants.

The national, 18-month HEJA 2010 study entailed two general phases: (a) instrument development and (b) implementation (i.e., data collection and analysis) (Doyle et al., 2012). The instrument development phase included in-depth interviews of subject matter experts, independent reviews by representatives of diverse health education work settings, and a modified Delphi approach through which task force members systematically integrated the interview and review outcomes into instrument development. A pilot survey resulted in further instrument refinement, subsequent revision and approval by an Institutional Review Board, and conduct of the first SOPHE/NCHEC online survey of job competencies and knowledge areas. The resulting updated model from the psychometric study, HEJA 2010, included Seven Areas of Responsibility, 34 Competencies, and 223 Sub-competencies (NCHEC, SOPHE, & AAHE, 2010). The three distinct levels of practice established through the CUP study were re-verified in the HEJA 2010 study based on extensive statistical analysis and professional judgment. The HEJA 2010 Model also included a hierarchy of entry-, advanced 1-, and advanced 2-level Sub-competencies.

The HEJA 2010 Steering Committee made recommendations for implementation of the HEJA 2010 results, which were endorsed by the CNHEO and the National Implementation Task Force for Accreditation in Health Education. The four recommendations were based on the previous recommendations, the SOPHE/AAHE National Task Force on Quality Assurance in Health Education's recommendations (Airhihenbuwa et al., 2005) and the CUP results. The steering committee recommended that: (a) appropriate levels of Sub-competencies be used in professional preparation programs, (b) NCHEC use the entry-level Sub-competencies for the CHES® certification examination, (c) NCHEC use both the entry- and advanced-level Sub-competencies for the certification examination for the new Master Certified Health Education Specialist (MCHES®) credential, and (d) all Sub-competencies be used for professional development activities. Multiple professional publications and presentations via webinars, face-to-face workshops and meetings were conducted by SOPHE and other CNHEO members during subsequent years to integrate the study findings into professional preparation and practice of health educators.

HEALTH EDUCATION SPECIALIST PRACTICE ANALYSIS I 2015 (HESPA I 2015)

As with the three-prior job/practice analyses, the HESPA I 2015 was undertaken to continue to build the foundation for quality assurance and to align the practice of health education with contemporary social and policy changes (e.g. emergence of social media, Affordable Care Act). The 18-month study was led by a steering committee (HESPA I 2015 SC) composed of the executive officers of NCHEC and SOPHE, the HEJA 2010 Task Force chair, and the HESPA I 2015 Task Force co-chairs, Drs. James McKenzie and Dixie Dennis, who were appointed by NCHEC and SOPHE. The HESPA I 2015 SC partnered with a 10-member HESPA I 2015 Task Force (HESPA I 2015 TF) composed of volunteer health education specialists who responded to a national invitation and were chosen from diverse practice settings, and practice analysis experts from Professional Examination Service (ProExam). Similar to HEJA 2010, the methods used to conduct HESPA I 2015 complied with credentialing industry standards and best-practice guidelines established by the National Commission of Certifying Agencies (ICE, 2014).

The HESPA I 2015 study comprised two phases. The first was the development of two validated data collection instruments: one instrument was created to collect ratings of Sub-competencies (i.e., skills) and the other to collect ratings of Knowledge items (See section VI). Two instruments were created to minimize the risk of fatigue from completing one long instrument. Content for both instruments was validated using an eight-step process that included input from a variety of certified and non-certified health education specialists. A pilot study of both instruments provided further refinement. The reliability of the data collected was established using interclass correlation coefficients. (Note: Information about the creation of the HESPA I 2015 instruments can be found in McKenzie et al., 2015). The results of the study re-verified three distinct levels of practice and yielded the updated HESPA I 2015 Model that included Seven Areas of Responsibility, 36 Competencies, and 258 Sub-competencies. Of the Sub-competencies, 141 were identified as Entry-level practice, 76 were Advanced 1-level practice, and 41 were Advanced 2-level practice. In addition, 131 Knowledge items were verified.

As in previous job/practice analyses, the HESPA I 2015 SC made recommendations for the implementation of the study results. They included: (1) creating and updating curricula for professional preparation programs at the undergraduate and graduate levels in health education/promotion; (2) updating the standards that form the basis for accreditation of professional preparation programs in health education; (3) updating the CHES® and MCHES® examinations to ensure that the examinations reflected contempo-

rary, realistic, and everyday practice; (4) planning and offering continuing education opportunities that were meaningful and helped health education professionals to strengthen their research and practice; (5) hiring health education specialists and developing job descriptions based on the HESPA I 2015 results; (6) conducting additional research on doctoral competencies for the health education profession; and (7) cross-walking the competencies of health education specialists with other public health and allied health professions to identify areas of similarities and differences. These recommendations were implemented by NCHEC and SOPHE, and members of the health education profession, over ensuing years.

IMPLICATIONS OF REVALIDATION OF COMPETENCIES STUDIES ON INDIVIDUAL CERTIFICATION

The results of previous studies that have revalidated Health Education Specialist Competencies have impacted individual certification and professional preparation and practice. The dissemination and endorsement of the CUP Model initiated changes to the structure of the CHES® examination for entry-level health education specialists. NCHEC leaders updated the CHES® examination blueprint framework for the certification examination questions, released a new study guide (NCHEC, 2007), and launched the first CHES® examination based on the CUP Model in fall, 2007. Performance pass rates on the new examination were comparable to previous performance pass rates (Dennis & Mahoney, 2008). These comparable performance pass rates validated that the primary components of the CUP Model not only reflected contemporary practice but also the professional preparation programs that are shaped by contemporary practice.

CUP findings regarding advanced-levels of practice also held significant implications for NCHEC and the profession. Following further discussions with multiple national leadership groups, there was broad consensus on creating distinct levels of certification between entry- and advanced-level certification. These factors and feasibility deliberations among various NCHEC working groups subsequently led NCHEC leaders to announce plans to develop an advanced-level of certification in the fall of 2008. In May 2009, following a period of public comment about such issues as eligibility criteria and certification mechanisms, the NCHEC Board of Commissioners issued a policy statement regarding the future availability of a new advanced-level credential (NCHEC, 2009). This statement revealed that the name of the certification was Master Certified Health Education Specialist (MCHES®) and included that eligibility for MCHES® was five years of experience, with certification based on a combination of entry- and advanced-level Competencies and Sub-competencies.

Following the completion of the HEJA 2010 Model and the HESPA I 2015 confirming an updated model of entry- and advanced-levels, the results were used to create a revised examination for CHES®. The advanced-level Sub-competencies were used in the Experience Documentation Opportunity (2010-2011) for current CHES®, which led to the MCHES® credential first being awarded in April 2011 (Chaney et al., 2013; Wilson et al., 2012). The inaugural MCHES® examination was administered in October 2011 (Dennis et al., 2012).

The results of HEJA 2010 were also used to establish professional development standards for those holding the MCHES® credential. These standards were revised to ensure that continuing education opportunities were in alignment with contemporary practice as outlined in HESPA I 2015 and then again after HESPA II 2020. CHES® and MCHES® individuals must accrue 75 continuing education contact hours in five years to maintain certification. Of the 75 hours, MCHES® must acquire 30 advanced-level hours related to advanced-level Sub-competencies.

In addition, the concept of continuing competence was adopted by NCHEC in 2019 in accordance with national and international accreditation standards (ICE, 2016; ISO/IEC, 2012) for certifying bodies. The change is intended to assist with meeting public expectations about the competence of practitioners in the field of health education and promotion. According to the *NCHEC Policies and Procedures Handbook*,

> Continuing Competency entails the demonstration of specified levels of knowledge, skills, or ability not only at the time of initial certification but throughout an individual's professional career. The NCHEC recertification requirements demonstrate the Continuing Competency of a Certified or Master Certified Health Education Specialist, as well as demonstrating a career commitment to the professional development and growth that represents an NCHEC credential (NCHEC, 2019, p.1).

Like all continuing education activities used to meet recertification requirements, Continuing Competency activities must be linked to the current validated Areas of Responsibility, Competencies, and Sub-competencies.

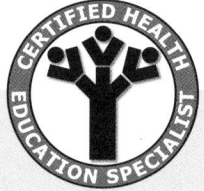

A Certified Health Education Specialist (CHES®) is an individual that has:

✓ met required academic preparation qualifications

✓ successfully passed a Competency-based examination administered by the National Commission for Health Education Credentialing, Inc.

✓ satisfies the continuing education requirement to maintain the national credential

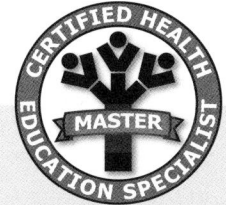

A Master Certified Health Education Specialist (MCHES ®) is an advanced-level practitioner that has:

✓ met required academic qualifications, worked in the field for a minimum of five years

✓ successfully passed a Competency-based examination administered by the National Commission for Health Education Credentialing, Inc.

✓ satisfies the continuing education requirement to maintain the national credential

ACCREDITATION OF THE CHES® AND MCHES® CERTIFICATION PROGRAMS

The CHES® and MCHES® certification programs were granted accreditation by the National Commission for Certifying Agencies (NCCA) in 2008 and 2013 respectively. The NCCA is the body of the Institute for Credentialing Excellence (ICE) that accredits professional certification organizations (ICE, 2009).

Obtaining the initial recognition of CHES®/MCHES® programs by this organization in testing accreditation made a profound statement within the national credentialing industry about the quality of the CHES®/MCHES® examinations. It is an additional characteristic of excellence of a clearly defined profession (Livingood & Auld, 2001; NCHEC, 2008). In 2018, the CHES®/MCHES® certification programs were granted reaccreditation.

In 2015, NCHEC earned the ISO 17024 accreditation as a Personnel Certification Body issued by the International Accreditation Service (IAS). This accreditation provides a global benchmark for personnel certification programs to ensure consistent, comparable and reliable operations worldwide. Obtaining the ISO 17024 accreditation is a confirmation that NCHEC's processes and systems align with acceptable global standards for personnel certifying organizations (IAS, n.d.).

Among the NCCA and IAS Standards for the Accreditation of Certification Programs, it is required that a professional role delineation or job analysis be conducted and periodically validated (ICE, 2016). To ensure that the content of NCHEC examinations reflects current practice in the profession and meets certification program accreditation standards, NCHEC committed to conducting job analyses every five years and continues to work with SOPHE in these efforts. In keeping with the five-year cycle, after HEJA 2010 and HESPA I 2015, the HESPA II 2020 began in February 2018 and concluded in August 2019 with dissemination in 2020. Thus, the accreditation standards for certifying agencies have had a critical impact on the progress of the health education profession.

COMPETENCY-BASED ACADEMIC PROGRAM ACCREDITATION

Various issues facing the profession in quality assurance, including a fragmented system of program approval processes and accreditation mechanisms, were addressed in 2000 by AAHE and SOPHE with an invitational meeting of key health education leaders. As a result, the National Task Force on Accreditation in Heath Education was convened by AAHE and SOPHE from 2001 to 2003. The Task Force was charged with developing a detailed plan for a coordinated accreditation system for baccalaureate and graduate programs in health education. The Task Force findings and recommendations laid the foundation for high-quality professional preparation and practice standards in health education. The findings and recommendations also provided strategic direction related to accreditation of community and school heath education preservice programs and individual credentialing (Allegrante et al., 2004).

A critical recommendation from the Task Force was that "a comprehensive, coordinated accreditation system for undergraduate and graduate health education should be put into place, which builds on the strengths of current mechanisms." (Allegrante et al., 2004, p. 672). Subsequently, between 2001 and 2003 the National Task Force on Accreditation in Health Education developed principles and seven recommendations for strengthening accreditation in health education which also impacted professional preparation and certification. In 2004, AAHE and SOPHE commissioned a new task force, the National Transition Task Force on Accreditation in Health Education, to help implement the recommendations between 2004 and 2006. In 2006, this Task Force convened the Third National Congress for Institutions Preparing Health Educators: Linking Program Assessment, Accountability, and Improvement, in Dallas, Texas a landmark meeting sometimes referred to as Dallas II. This conference was referred to as Dallas II because the earlier congress of 1996, which was designed for attendees to discuss graduate-level Competencies, was also held in Dallas (the first congress was in Birmingham, Alabama, in 1981) (Taub, et al., 2009).

The Dallas II meeting, sponsored by SOPHE and AAHE, drew together approximately 250 university faculty members and administrators from over 150 professional preparation programs (Taub et al., 2009), as well as practitioners. The purpose of Dallas II was to provide an update of the effort to establish a unified system of accreditation for the health education profession, review and discuss future accreditation developments, disseminate and discuss the implications of the new CUP Model, and identify issues and strategies for the transition to a unified accreditation system.

According to Taub et al. (2009), accreditation discussions focused on potential avenues for transitioning to a more coordinated system. Since 1988, AAHE had partnered with the National Council for Accreditation of Teacher Education (NCATE), the recognized accrediting body for professional preparation programs in school health education. The Council on Education for Public Health (CEPH) had been accrediting master's level programs and schools of public health since 1974 (a process originally established by health education leaders and maintained by the American Public Health Association since the early 1940s). In 1980, SOPHE established an approval process for baccalaureate public or community health education programs, and in 1984 AAHE joined to form the SOPHE/AAHE Baccalaureate Program Approval Committee (SABPAC). SABPAC approval was based on the Competencies of health education specialists and included a peer-review process using self-study assessment criteria. However, the lack of an official accreditation designation for the SABPAC was a challenge (Capwell, et al., 2019). In 2005, CEPH began to accredit baccalaureate public or community health education programs linked to graduate public health programs and schools but did not accredit standalone baccalaureate public or community health education programs (CEPH, 2005).

A part of the Dallas II discussions revolved around the possibility of CEPH becoming the accrediting body for all professional preparation programs in community health education, regardless of their affiliation status with graduate-level public health schools and programs (Taub et al., 2009). Attendees discussed challenges as they related to differences in terminology regarding a "unified" versus a "coordinated" multiple body accrediting system, potential philosophical differences between public and community health, and capacity challenges for small professional preparation programs that needed to be accredited.

Dallas II attendees deemed further exploration into accreditation possibilities important. Following the Dallas II meeting, SOPHE and AAHE established the

Section I: Historical Perspectives

National Implementation Task Force for Accreditation in Health Education in 2007 to continue the momentum of the National Transition Task Force in pursuing a coordinated accreditation system (Cottrell et al., 2009). Meanwhile, SOPHE and AAHE integrated the Areas of Responsibility, Competencies, and Sub-competencies from the CUP findings into the SABPAC approval requirements (SOPHE & AAHE, 2007). For CEPH leaders and other stakeholders, the CUP Model and the results of any future role delineation research needed to be an essential part of future accreditation discussions (Taub et al., 2009). Unifying the profession on accreditation for professional preparation required a unanimous acceptance and application of the current Areas of Responsibility, Competencies, and Sub-competencies as the basis for individual certification and health education practice.

Beginning in 2007, CEPH began to explore the possibility of accrediting baccalaureate public health programs, including those in community or public health education even when they were not administered in conjunction with a CEPH-accredited graduate-level program. After gathering input from various stakeholders and obtaining specific advice from a group of thought leaders in 2011, CEPH decided to develop accreditation criteria for standalone baccalaureate public health programs (SBPs). CEPH determined that the accreditation opportunity would be available to all baccalaureate public health programs, not only those with a concentration in public or community health education (Cottrell, et al., 2012). Between 2011 and 2013, CEPH developed, vetted, and revised criteria and procedures to accredit SBPs (Figueroa, et al., 2015). During this time, the National Implementation Task Force on Accreditation in Health Education continued to update and provide guidance to professional preparation programs in health education to prepare for CEPH accreditation.

CEPH criteria for SBPs were adopted in June 2013, and CEPH accepted its first nine applications for SBP accreditation in February 2014. In a pilot study in 2014, two community health education programs mapped their curricula to both the public health core described in the CEPH criteria and the NCHEC Competencies. Figueroa, et al., (2015) found the content and skills to be complementary and the overlap substantial enough to ensure that specialty content in community health education would not be sacrificed in the new accreditation system.

In June 2016, the first four public health SBP's were accredited by CEPH. At the time of this writing, there were 13 accredited SBP's (CEPH, 2019a) and 14 more moving through the accreditation process (CEPH, 2019b). These numbers do not include those undergraduate public health programs that are accredited as part of a school or program of public health. Once the accreditation process for SBPs began, the SABPAC approval process was officially phased out in 2014.

In the last decade, there have also been significant changes in accreditation of professional preparation programs for school health educators (Taub et al., 2014). Historically, the United States Department of Education and the Council for Higher Education Accreditation have recognized two organizations as professional accrediting bodies for teacher preparation: The National Council for Accreditation of Teacher Education (NCATE) and the Teacher Education Accreditation Council (TEAC). As of July 1, 2013, NCATE and TEAC consolidated to become the Council for the Accreditation of Educator Preparation (TEAC, 2014; CAEP, 2015). The creation of CAEP provided an opportunity to create a unified accreditation system that strengthens the performance standards of teacher education candidates, raises the stature of the teaching profession, and improves the standards for the evidence that supports claims of quality (Taub et al., 2014). Until June 2019, the Society of Health and Physical Educators (SHAPE) was recognized by CAEP as the Specialized Professional Association (SPA) in health education. In fall 2019, SOPHE was approved by CAEP to become the health education SPA based on the HESPA II 2020 results (S. Goekler & A. Lyde Gabrielson, personal communication, September 23, 2018).

MOVING FORWARD: CONTINUED GROWTH AND CHANGE

In addition to creating advanced-level certification and achieving NCCA and IAS accreditation for the CHES® and MCHES® certification programs, and as noted in Figure 1.1, the health education profession has continued to grow and evolve since the 1970s. The United States Department of Labor (USDOL) recognized "health educator" as a distinct standard occupational classification in 2000 (Office of Management and Budget, 2000) and predicted the occupation to grow faster than other occupations (USDOL, 2018). In 2015, due to a SOPHE and NCHEC appeal, the Department of Labor agreed to modify the classification title (21-1091) to "health education specialist" (J. Chi, personal communication, July 23, 2018). Employers have increasingly included CHES®/MCHES® "preferred" or "required" in job descriptions (Cottrell et al., 2012). Efforts have been undertaken to develop a global set of Competencies for health promotion professionals (Allegrante et al., 2009; Allegrante et al., 2012), while passage of the Patient Protection and Affordable Care Act in 2010 further catalyzed interest in the domestic role of health education specialists in disease prevention and health promotion (Auld, 2017; Bruening et al, 2018).

Developments in reimbursement for health education services under the direction of a physician may provide additional employment opportunities for health education specialists (Chambliss et al., 2014). Baccalaureate and graduate programs in public health have grown significantly in recent decades, with concomitant changes in accreditation and quality assurance systems affecting health education (Cottrell et al., 2012). Additionally, various social, political and environmental changes have drastically impacted health

education research and practice (e.g. technological innovations with eHealth, mHealth and social media, evidence-based approach related to the impact of policy/systems changes on individual and population health) (Allegrante & Auld, 2019; Bruening et al., 2018). Such changes command new knowledge and skills of health education specialists to be effective moving forward.

It remains critically important to perform periodic practice analyses to adequately assess changing knowledge and skills for health education practice. This concept is supported by part of the CNHEO's profession-wide strategic plan which specifies the need to continue strengthening professional preparation, professional development and credentialing, including the objective to "cooperate with the on-going practice analysis conducted every 5 years for health education specialists" (CNHEO, 2018, p.3).

The HEPSA II 2020 resulted in the adjustment to Eight Areas of Responsibility by separating Ethics and Professionalism into a separate Area of Responsibility rather than interspersed within other Areas of Responsibility. Also, the splitting of Communications and Advocacy into separate Areas of Responsibility is reflective of the rapid expansion of communication strategies and technology and acknowledging the increased emphasis of advocacy to effectively address the socio-ecologic factors impacting the health of individuals, communities, and populations (Allegrante & Auld, 2019; Bruening et al., 2018). Undoubtedly, unfolding evolutionary changes in genome discovery, social determinants of health, cross-sector collaboration, and other areas to name just a few, underscore the invaluable need for continued psychometric studies of the knowledge and skills needed by future health education specialists and the requisite role of SOPHE, NCHEC and other health education allies in meeting their needs.

FIGURE 1.1: Historical Timeline of Selected Milestones

	1967	1969	1972	1978	1985	1987
Role Delineation/ Framework Adaptations	Society for Public Health Education (SOPHE) published Statement of Functions of Community Health Educators and Minimum Requirements for their Professional Preparation			Role Delineation Project began *Helen P. Cleary*	Original Entry-level Competency Framework completed	SOPHE and AAHE joined forces to operate the Society for Public Health Education and American Association for Health Education Baccalaureate Program Approval Committee (SABPAC)
Program Accreditation and Approvals		American Public Health Association (APHA) published Criteria and Guidelines for Accrediting Graduate Programs in Community Health Education	Association for Advancement in Health Education (AAHE) began conducting portfolio reviews under National Council for Accreditation of Teacher Education (NCATE)	SOPHE initiated an approval process for baccalaureate community health programs		

	1988	1989	1990	1992	1998	2001
Role Delineation/ Framework Adaptations				Joint Committee for graduate standards created	National Health Educator Competencies Update Project (CUP) initiated *CUP Key Leaders*	
Professional Certification	National Commission for Health Education Credentialing, Inc. (NCHEC) established	First chartered Certified Health Education Specialists	First CHES® exam offered			
Program Accreditation and Approvals			NCHEC continuing education/professional development system established			National Taskforce on Accreditation in Health Education established

	2004	2005	2006	2007	2008	2010
Role Delineation/ Framework Adaptations			CUP model adopted *2006*		Health Educator Job Analysis (HEJA) initiated	HEJA model adopted
Professional Certification				CUP-based CHES® exam offered	CHES® program accredited by National Commission for Certifying Agencies (NCCA)	HEJA-based Master Certified Health Education Specialist (MCHES®) Early Documentation Opportunity (EDO) initiated
Program Accreditation and Approvals	National Transition Task Force on Accreditation in Health Education established	Council on Education for Public Heath (CEPH) accreditation standards for baccalaureate programs of public health schools/ programs created	National Implementation Task Force on Accreditation in Health Education established & convened Third National Congress for Institutions Preparing Health Educators	SABPAC integrated CUP model into requirements	*HEJA 2010 panel*	*2010*

Section I: Historical Perspectives

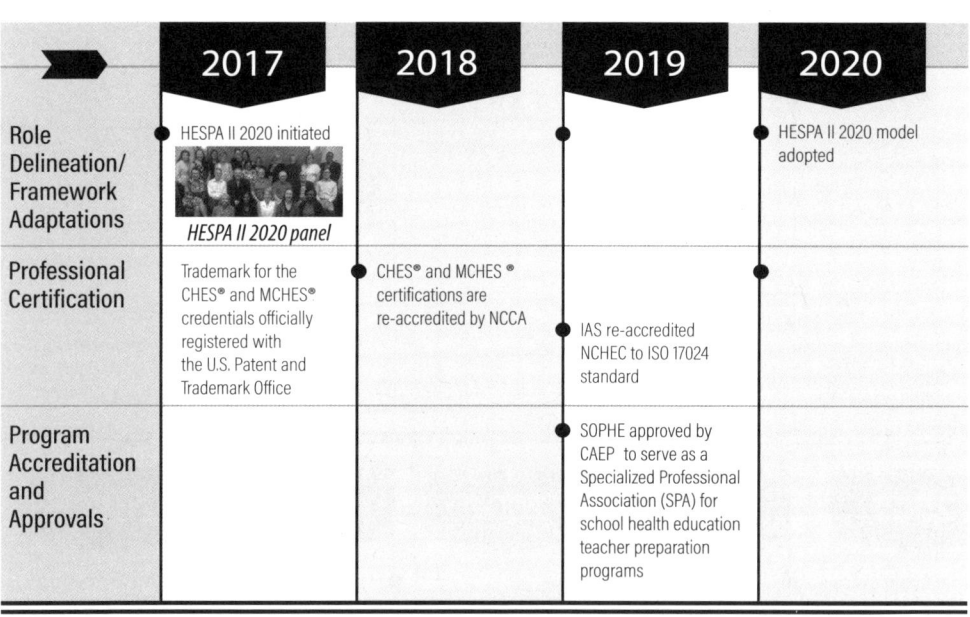

	2011	2012	2013	2014	2015	2016
Role Delineation/ Framework Adaptations			HESPA I 2015 initiated		HESPA I 2015 model adopted	
Professional Certification	• MCHES® EDO completed • First MCHES® exam offered	HEJA-based CHES® exam offered	CHES® certification is re-accredited and MCHES® certification accredited by the National Commission for Certifying Agencies (NCCA)		International Accreditation Service (IAS) accredited NCHEC to ISO 17024 standard	HESPA I-based CHES® and MCHES ® exams offered
Program Accreditation and Approvals	The National Transition Task Force on Accreditation in Health Education requested CEPH accredit free-standing undergraduate public health programs		CEPH accreditation standards for standalone baccalaureate programs in public health created	NCATE & Teacher Education Accreditation Council (TEAC) consolidated to become Council for the Accreditation of Educator Preparation (CAEP) • AAHE sunsetted • SABPAC sunsetted	*2015*	CEPH accredited first undergraduate public health programs

	2017	2018	2019	2020
Role Delineation/ Framework Adaptations	HESPA II 2020 initiated *HESPA II 2020 panel*			HESPA II 2020 model adopted
Professional Certification	Trademark for the CHES® and MCHES® credentials officially registered with the U.S. Patent and Trademark Office	CHES® and MCHES ® certifications are re-accredited by NCCA	IAS re-accredited NCHEC to ISO 17024 standard	
Program Accreditation and Approvals			SOPHE approved by CAEP to serve as a Specialized Professional Association (SPA) for school health education teacher preparation programs	

Section II   HESPA II 2020 Process and Outcomes

The Health Education Specialist Practice Analysis II 2020 (HESPA II 2020) was conducted to revalidate the contemporary practice of entry- and advanced-level health education specialists. The findings will be used to develop updated examinations for Certified Health Education Specialists (CHES®) and Master Certified Health Education Specialists (MCHES®), as well as to report validated changes in health education practice since the HESPA I 2015. The HESPA II 2020 will also inform professional preparation and continuing education initiatives. This study was initiated in 2017 to meet accreditation standards of the National Commission for Certifying Agencies (NCCA), which requires a regular revalidation of the Competencies upon which the credential is based.

Practice analysis experts from Scantron oversaw the HESPA II 2020 study. Scantron adhered to the highest credentialing industry standards as outlined in federal regulation (*Uniform Guidelines on Employee Selection Procedures*) and manuals, such as *Standards for Educational and Psychological Testing* (American Educational Research Association, 2014). Scantron staff employed these standards as well as the National Commission for Certifying Agencies *Standards for the Accreditation of Certification Programs* (ICE, 2014, 2016) and the International Organization for Standardization/International Electrotechnical Commission (ISO/IEC) 17024 (2012) throughout the study.

The HESPA II 2020 study was guided by the principle that "health education is a single profession, with common roles and responsibilities" (Allegrante et al., 2004, p. 676). The processes used in this study were built on the work of previous research studies in this field, the Role Delineation Project (Cleary, 1995), CUP (Gilmore et al., 2005), HEJA 2010 (Doyle et al., 2012), and HESPA I 2015 (McKenzie et al, 2016).

HESPA II 2020 PARTICIPANTS

Under the direction of Scantron, the Health Education Specialist Practice Analysis II 2020 (HESPA II 2020) Technical Advisory Group (TAG) led the study with essential input from the HESPA II 2020 Health Education Practice Panel (HEPP). The TAG consisted of the chief staff officers from each sponsoring organization (NCHEC and SOPHE), the co-chair of HESPA I 2015, the HESPA II 2020 chair and vice-chair appointed by NCHEC and SOPHE, the coordinator for the Division Board for Certified Health Education Specialists (DBCHES), and an NCHEC staff person. The TAG and Scantron employees publicized a *call to the profession* to assist with the study that generated a pool of 143 volunteer nominees. From the pool of volunteers, the TAG selected 17 individuals to serve on the HEPP who were diverse along variables that affect the practice of health education including work setting, experience level, educational background, demographic groups, and geographic settings. The volunteers agreed to participate in several conference calls and three in-person meetings, for which their travel was reimbursed. The HEPP examined the Responsibilities, Competencies, and Sub-Competencies that eventually became the basis for the survey instrument that was developed by the TAG and Scantron. The volunteer pool was also used to recruit individuals to pilot test the survey instruments.

Recruitment of Survey Participants

Two primary goals guided the recruitment of survey participants: (1) to involve as many health education specialists (both certified and non-certified) as possible and (2) to achieve representation from all work settings, education levels, years of experience, and health education certification statuses. Because there exists no single data source for the entire group of practicing health education specialists, multiple approaches were used to invite as many health education specialists as possible to participate. In an effort to reach broadly into the profession, NCHEC and SOPHE staff members identified some 200 contacts at health education organizations, including member organizations of the Coalition of National Health Education Organizations (CNHEO) and national and state affiliates of major health education associations responsible for electronic mailing lists. Each of these contacts received an e-mail and/or personal telephone call to request organizational assistance in publicizing the study and to provide an invitation and link to the online survey registration form for their mailing lists. The identified groups participated in various capacities in advertising the study, including e-mailing information to their mailing lists and posting announcements on their Web sites and/or on social media handles.

NCHEC and SOPHE staff members created Internet banners hyperlinked to the survey instrument to advertise the study on their Web sites and on social media. The hyperlinked images were also used as part of their e-mail signatures. The staff members of both organizations also collaborated on a special social media hash tag: #HESPA II 2020. NCHEC and SOPHE employed this hash tag for survey announcements posted via Twitter and Facebook. Staff members encouraged survey participation continually through announcements at various conferences throughout the survey period.

The next step of the sampling strategy was to invite all national and chapter SOPHE members and all individuals holding CHES® and MCHES® certification to participate in the survey using e-mail addresses provided by SOPHE and NCHEC and sent when the survey opened on November 5, 2018. The NCHEC and SOPHE lists were combined into a single list and duplicates removed. The combined list included 13,271 individuals. One Continuing Education Contact Hour (CECH) was offered as an incentive for CHES®

and MCHES® certificants if they completed the survey. Another optional incentive for all who completed the survey was a drawing for one of twenty gift cards in the amount of $50. NCHEC and SOPHE both placed information about the survey prominently on their Web sites with a link to the survey landing page.

HESPA II 2020 PROCEDURES

The HESPA II 2020 study spanned 22 months from October 2017 to August 2019. During this period, those who conducted the study selected volunteers as previously described, developed survey instruments and collected, analyzed, and interpreted data. Typically, a practice analysis includes two major implementation phases, the first of which is the development of a model of Areas of Responsibility, Competencies, Sub-competencies, and Knowledge, and the second of which is a validation study. Adding the steps for advanced planning and communication of results, the entire process consisted of five phases (see Figure 2.1).

Conceptual Framework for Instrument Development

As illustrated in Figure 2.1, the TAG and Scantron personnel played a critical role throughout the practice analysis. The HEPP's work began with a review of the HESPA I 2015 Framework and Knowledge list. From there, the HEPP reviewed three relevant articles (Bruening, et al., 2018; McKenzie et al., 2016; National Commission for Health Education Credentialing, Inc., 2015) identified by the TAG in advance of the first in-person meeting to help orient panelists to the breadth of perspectives needed for the practice analysis meetings.

In reviewing the 2015 hierarchical model, the HEPP agreed that the number of Sub-competencies was high (258) and that it would be desirable to synthesize these statements for the new outline. The HEPP reviewed the definitions of the priority populations

Section II: HESPA II 2020 Process and Outcomes

FIGURE 2.1: *HESPA II 2020: Five Phases*

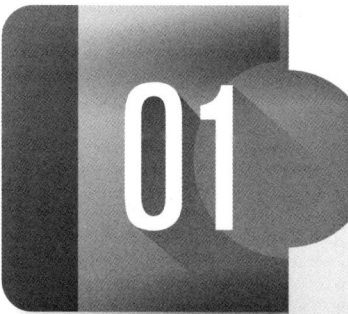

Planning
October 2017 - May 2018

1. *Partner Planning:* Study Sponsors SOPHE and NCHEC leadership make initial plans for next Practice Analysis.
2. *Selection of Project Leadership:* Chair and Vice Chair and the practice analysis leadership group called the Technical Advisory Group (TAG).
3. *Request for Proposal disseminated, contract awarded:* Castle/Scantron, selected.
4. *Consultation with previous job/practice analysis study leaders:* Call with TAG.
5. *TAG Planning Meetings (14 conference calls):* Develop research questions and process.
6. *Call for Health Education Practice Panel Volunteers:* Public call and then application review and selection by TAG.

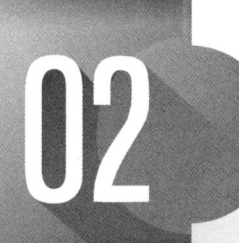

Development and Refinement of the Areas of Responsibility, Competencies, and Sub-competencies
May-July 2018

1. *HEPP working meetings:* Three in-person meetings for a total of eight full days.
   a. Meeting 1: Brainstorming session on the current responsibilities of health education specialists, approval of definitions and research questions, review of current model, reached consensus on Areas of Responsibility.
   b. Meeting 2: Small group work on Competencies and Sub-competencies. Addressed synthesis of related statements to reduce numbers.
   c. Meeting 3: Review Sub-competencies, draft Knowledge items.
2. *Final Review of Areas of Responsibility, Competencies, and Sub-competencies by TAG:* Via e-mail and 2 conference calls.

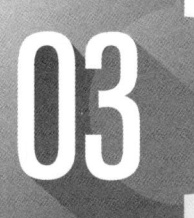

Data Collection
July 2018-January 2019

1. *Sampling plan development (2 conference calls):* Development of a sampling plan for the validation survey by Scantron and outreach to the profession for volunteer survey via e-mail and conference calls.
2. *Creation of Survey instrument (14 conference calls):* TAG and Scantron via e-mail and conference calls.
3. *Institutional Review Board approval:* Approval of the study by the Institutional Review Board of the University of Alabama.
4. *Instrument pilot:* Pilot testing of the online survey instrument for comprehensiveness, clarity, and technical ease of use.
5. *Participant sampling:* E-mail invitations to participate in the survey sent to health education specialists followed by periodic reminders sent throughout a three-month completion window. Postcards to those who had not completed survey plus APHA members of sections PHEHP and SHES.

Data Analysis and Acceptance
February 2019-August 2019

1. *Data Analysis* (February-July 2019)
   a. Scantron conducted a series of statistical analyses of survey responses.
   b. Scantron and TAG met in-person.
   c. TAG electronic review via conference calls (20) and e-mail reviews.
2. *Model finalization*
   a. Technical Report from Scantron.
   b. Acceptance of report by SOPHE and NCHEC boards.

Communication and Utilization of Results
September 2019 forward

1. *Report to the Profession*
   a. Series of Recommendations for the Profession accepted by SOPHE and NCHEC boards regarding use of report.
   b. Series of Recommendations for the Profession accepted by CNHEO.
   c. Presentation at major health education conferences and webinars.
   d. Develop Framework & Companion Guide.
   e. Update NCHEC exams.

Section II: HESPA II 2020 Process and Outcomes

FIGURE 2.2: *HESPA II 2020 Timeline*

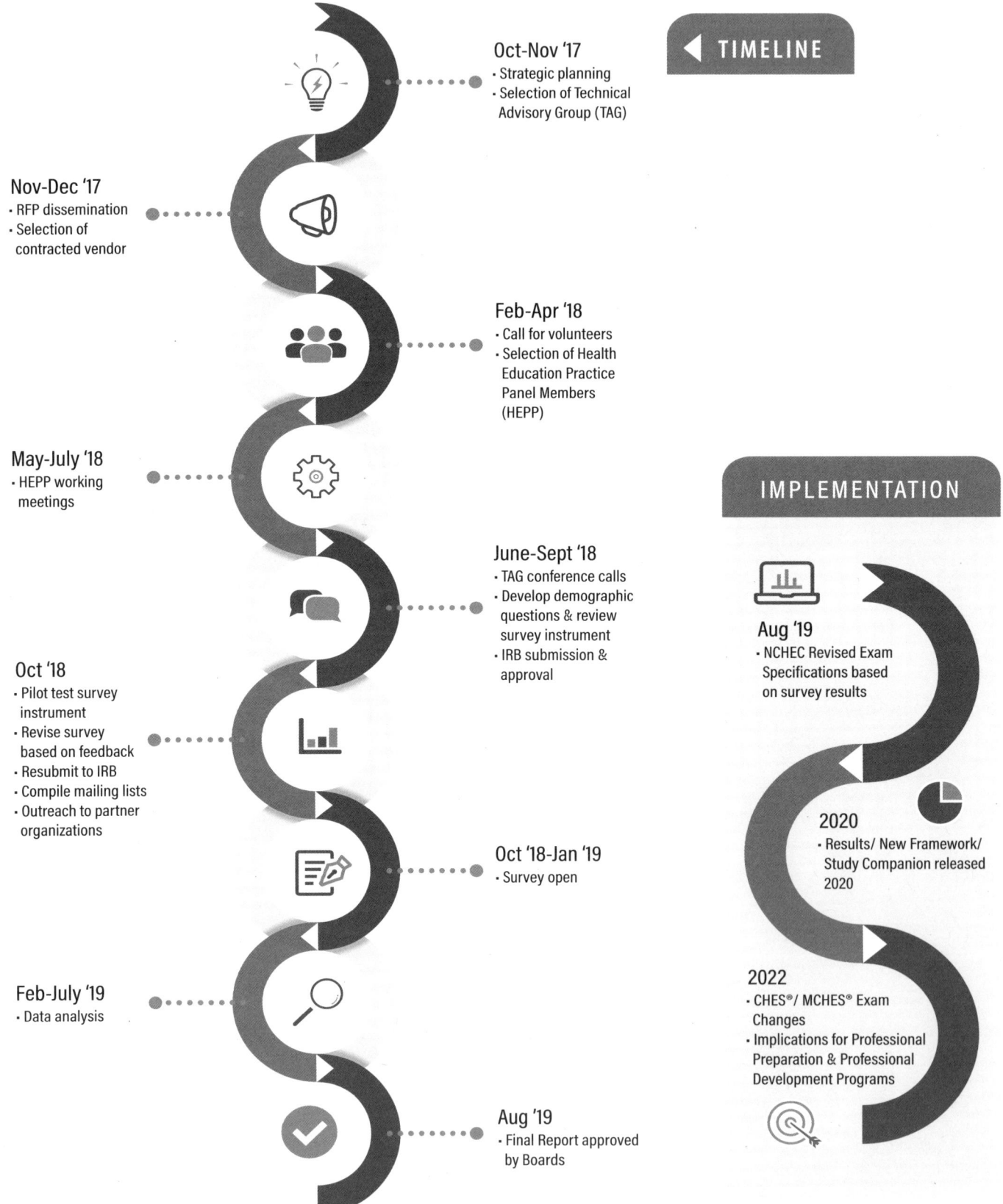

Oct-Nov '17
- Strategic planning
- Selection of Technical Advisory Group (TAG)

Nov-Dec '17
- RFP dissemination
- Selection of contracted vendor

Feb-Apr '18
- Call for volunteers
- Selection of Health Education Practice Panel Members (HEPP)

May-July '18
- HEPP working meetings

June-Sept '18
- TAG conference calls
- Develop demographic questions & review survey instrument
- IRB submission & approval

Oct '18
- Pilot test survey instrument
- Revise survey based on feedback
- Resubmit to IRB
- Compile mailing lists
- Outreach to partner organizations

Oct '18-Jan '19
- Survey open

Feb-July '19
- Data analysis

Aug '19
- Final Report approved by Boards

TIMELINE

IMPLEMENTATION

Aug '19
- NCHEC Revised Exam Specifications based on survey results

2020
- Results/ New Framework/ Study Companion released 2020

2022
- CHES®/ MCHES® Exam Changes
- Implications for Professional Preparation & Professional Development Programs

and then reached consensus on minor suggestions for revision. After this discussion, panelists expressed clear understanding that the purpose of the practice analysis was to address the breadth of the health education profession but complete mastery of every Competency is not expected.

The HEPP then focused on the existing hierarchical model, in place since 2015, and the updates that would ensure the new model's currency and adequacy for the upcoming five-year period. Through small group work and facilitated discussion, participants reached consensus in the first meeting on the Areas of Responsibility and Competencies that are appropriate for the health education specialists working at different levels, with different levels of education, and in a variety of practice settings. After considerable discussion, it was decided that the Seven Areas of Responsibility in the HESPA I 2015 model did not pro-vide enough emphasis on advocacy and that Ethics and Professionalism should be a separate Area of Responsibility instead of being integrated throughout all Responsibilities. As a result, the HEPP decided to add an eighth Area of Responsibility. Additionally, some of the Competencies were realigned under different Areas of Responsibility. From a professional preparation and professional development perspec-tive, the addition of the eighth Area of Responsibility does not create an entirely new area of preparation, but more a reprioritization and refocusing of existing Competencies and Sub-competencies. The Areas of Responsibility proposed by the HEPP are as follows:

- Assessment of Needs and Capacity
- Planning
- Implementation
- Evaluation and Research
- Advocacy
- Communication
- Leadership and Management
- Ethics and Professionalism

In the early stages of updating the Areas of Responsibility, Competencies, and Sub-competencies for use in the study, HEPP discussed the types and depth of knowledge that health education specialists needed to possess to effectively perform a specific Competency or Sub-competency. This topic arose most frequently during discussions regarding current practice and the long-range use of study outcomes to shape professional preparation and development efforts. Like the HESPA I 2015 Task Force members and the HEJA 2010 Task Force members before them, the HEPP agreed that a Competency-based approach to professional preparation, credentialing, and development was essential. Competencies from HESPA I 2015 were thoroughly reviewed. In some cases, similar Competencies were combined and where needed new Competencies were developed. The HEPP also acknowledged that while slightly different definitions were available, for use in this study the terms health education/promotion could be combined.

Next, panelists needed to determine the Sub-competencies for each Competency. The panelists worked in small groups; each having been assigned Competencies for which to write Sub-competencies. After the Sub-competencies had been drafted in small groups, the entire HEPP convened to review and refine them, a set of conversations that required the remainder of the second meeting. There was discussion about the number of Competencies and Sub-competencies that had been developed in 2015, and the HEPP negotiated ways to improve synthesis by reducing overlap and combining related statements. This strategy led to a reduction in the number of Competencies and Sub-competencies.

Also, as with HEJA 2010 and HESPA I 2015, the HEPP recognized the utility of identifying relevant Knowledge items to be included in professional preparation and continuing education programs. For this reason, the HEPP decided to collect survey data to again verify Knowledge items. The HEPP used similar procedures as used in the HEJA 2010 and HESPA I 2015 study to compose the 149 Knowledge items for the HESPA II 2020 survey. Therefore, the piloted instrument included 191 Sub-competency statements and 149 Knowledge items.

Survey Instrument

Utilizing the Responsibilities, Competencies, Sub-competencies and Knowledge items as determined by the HEPP, Scantron, with extensive input from the TAG, developed two draft survey instruments. One instrument focused on the Responsibilities, Competencies and Sub-competencies while the second instrument focused on the Responsibilities and Knowledge items.

NCHEC and SOPHE staff desired to adhere to best practice related to research with human participants. The Vice Chair of the TAG, who served on faculty at the University of Alabama, was instrumental in securing Institutional Review Board (IRB) approval for the project. The application for IRB approval was initially submitted on August 15, 2018 and final approval was granted on September 14, 2018, with an expiration of September 10, 2019.

After IRB approval had been granted, a pilot test of the survey was conducted. The purpose of the pilot test was to assess the clarity of directions, functionality of the survey driver, and the time required to complete the survey instruments. The pilot test sample (n = 25) was not intended to be representative of the field in any meaningful way; instead, participants were identified using the list of individuals who had expressed interest in serving on the HEPP but were not selected, augmented by a small number of others. Scantron invited the sample participants using an e-mail request sent on October 2, 2018, and managed data collection using reminder e-mails to boost participation by the deadline of October 15, 2018. Participation in the pilot test resulted in 13 completed and usable surveys (nine completed the Competency

surveys and four completed the Knowledge surveys). Following review of pilot survey responses, several changes were made to the survey instruments. An amended IRB application was submitted with the revised instrument on October 22, 2018. Final approval was granted by the University of Alabama IRB on November 5, 2018.

The TAG devoted much time to a discussion of the rating scales to be used in the survey. Ultimately the decision was made to use the same importance and frequency rating scales employed in the CUP, HEJA 2010, and HESPA I 2015 studies to permit comparisons of the HESPA II 2020 findings with those in the previous three studies. In addition, at the suggestion of Scantron experts, a performance expectation scale was added to this version. The scales differed slightly depending on how they were used in the survey instruments. The scales used in the Competency survey were as follows:

Importance: How important is the Area of Responsibility to your work as a health education specialist? OR How important are the Competencies and Sub-competencies in each Area of Responsibility to your work as a health education specialist?
    1 = Not Important
    2 = Minimally Important
    3 = Moderately Important
    4 = Highly Important

Frequency: On average, how frequently did you perform this activity in your work as a health education specialist during the past 12 months?
    1 = Not at all
    2 = Occasionally (less than once a month)
    3 = Frequently (at least once per month)
    4 = Very frequently (at least once per week)

Performance Expectation: At what point in your employment as a health education specialist were you first expected to perform the Area of Responsibility,

Competency, or Sub-competency?

0 = Never

1 = Year 1

2 = Year 2 through year 5

3 = After year 5

The scales were modified slightly for use in the Knowledge survey instrument, in that instead of Competency or Sub-competency, the scales referred to Knowledge items. After each series of questions, respondents were also given an open-ended opportunity to add any comments or areas that they thought were missing from the Competency or Knowledge items.

Development of the demographic portion of the survey instrument began with the questions that had been used in previous studies. These were reviewed and refined for the current project by Scantron staff and the TAG. For example, drawing on feedback received from respondents in HESPA I 2015, the TAG refined the work setting options available to respondents in this survey instrument. As negotiated by the TAG, the demographic survey addressed the respondent's preparation, experience, and practice as a health education specialist. The survey also included questions about basic personal characteristics of respondents such as age, ethnicity and race, and gender. As is generally recommended in survey development, the demographic questions were placed at the end of the instrument after the Competency or Knowledge items were completed. As a result of this decision, demographic information was not collected on anyone who completed only part of the survey.

Analysis and Outcomes

Scantron employees compiled survey responses, performed data analysis, and guided the TAG in the interpretation of the results. As a part of this work, Scantron employees: (a) developed demographic profiles of participants (group percentages) based on certification status (i.e., CHES® or MCHES® vs. non-certified, educational degrees earned, years of experience, and work setting and (b) developed subgroup analyses based upon work setting, years of experience, certification status, and education levels. The data analysis for this project was generated using SAS software, Version 9.4 of the SAS System for Windows.

The survey items were uploaded on a survey driver, which had been programmed in Cold Fusion 9.0. Counts and percentages were computed for most demographic questions.

Data were then divided into two groups: one made up of respondents who provided every rating requested in the survey (i.e., 702 ratings in the Competency survey and 320 ratings in the Knowledge survey); compared with a second group comprising every respondent who did not provide every rating in the survey. Scantron staff then performed a Principal Components Analysis to determine if the ratings provided by the two groups were homogeneous, or if there was a point of completion that could be identified as a threshold to use to eliminate responses. The eigenvalues derived from the Principal Components Analysis were then compared using a threshold of 1.0, indicating homogeneity and an analysis of variance (ANOVA), which determined there was no significant difference in ratings provided by the groups, for either the Competency survey ($p = 0.21$) or the Knowledge survey ($p = 0.61$). Therefore, all individuals completing any portion of the survey were included in the data analysis.

DEMOGRAPHICS

The 3,851 survey participants represented all 50 states, the District of Columbia, and Puerto Rico, while 31 respondents indicated they were working outside of the United States. The largest percentages of participants were from California (10.0%, n = 198), Texas (6.2%, n = 123), and New York (5.3%, n = 105). A majority of the participants identified as female (88.3%, n = 1,774), White (75.5%, n = 1,493), Non-Hispanic (87.3%, n = 1753 and the largest number of respondents fell within the 26 – 35 year age range (41.1%, n = 827). A majority also indicated that they worked full-time as defined in the survey as working 30 hours or more per week (80.6%, n =1,616). When asked about the highest degree earned, the majority of participants reported earning some type of master's degree. When more specifically asked about the highest degree earned with a health education emphasis, the majority of respondents still reported a master's degree, with over half of those being Master of Public Health (MPH) degrees (See Table 2.1).

Table 2.2 examines a number of professional characteristics associated with the survey participants. Certification status is the first variable examined and the majority of respondents who answered this question were either CHES® or MCHES® certified. In addition, 401 participants identified one or more other certifications. Of these, the most common certification was the Wellness Coach. The next aspect of the table considers the number of years of experience participants have had in health education; almost one-third of the respondents (30.9%) who answered the question have worked from zero to four years. The next largest experience range is five to nine years (24.3%). The majority of respondents have worked in their current position for one to four years (66.1%). Another way of looking at the data is that 83% of the respondents began their current employment within the last ten years. Less than 5% have held their current employment for more than 20 years. Finally, the table presents information on membership status in professional associations. Most participants who responded to this question belonged to SOPHE and/or APHA.

Participants were also asked to identify their work setting (See Table 2.3). Of the 3,851 participants, 2,011 indicated their primary work setting. The great-est percentage of participants identified their work setting as a Public Health Agency (22.9%, n = 461), followed by health care (18.0%, n = 361), academia (17.3%, n = 348), community (16.7%, n = 336), business/worksite (8.3%, n = 167), college health (5.5%, n = 110), other (6.6%, n = 132), and school health (4.1%, n = 82). The seven major categories of work reflect the range of settings where contemporary health education specialists work. The HESPA II 2020 respondents' current work settings align with the three prior job analysis studies.

Table: 2.1
Demographic Data of Survey Participants

Characteristics	n*	Percent
Gender		
Female	1774	88.3%
Male	210	10.5%
Other	3	0.1%
Prefer not to answer	21	1.0%
Total	**2008***	**100%**
Ethnicity: Hispanic, Latino or Spanish origin		
No, not of Hispanic, Latino, or Spanish origin	1753	87.3%
Yes, Mexican, Mexican American. or Chicano	92	4.6%
Yes, Puerto Rican	29	1.4%
Yes, Cuban	8	0.4%
Yes, another Hispanic Latino, or Spanish Origin	61	3.0%
Prefer not to answer	64	3.2%
Total	**2007***	**100%**

Characteristics	n*	Percent
Racial Background		
White	1493	75.5%
Black or African American	289	14.6%
American Indian or Alaska Native	24	1.2%
Asian Indian	21	1.1%
Japanese	10	0.5%
Native Hawaiian	5	0.3%
Chinese	24	1.2%
Korean	8	0.4%
Guamanian or Chamorro	1	0.1%
Filipino	36	1.8%
Vietnamese	4	0.2%
Samoan	1	0.1%
Other Asian	16	0.8%
Other Pacific Islander	1	0.1%
Some Other Race	44	2.2%
Total	**1977***	**100%**
Age		
Under 25	173	8.6%
26-35	827	41.1%
36-45	433	21.5%
46-55	270	13.4%
56-65	217	10.8%
66-75	59	2.9%
Over 75	3	0.1%
Prefer not to answer	28	1.4%
Total	**2010***	**100%**

Characteristics	n*	Percent
Employment Status		
Full-time (30 hours or more per week	1616	80.6%
Part-time (less than30 hours per week	390	19.4%
Total	**2006***	**100%**
Education (Highest level of education completed)		
Bachelors	354	17.6%
Some Post-bachelor's education	88	4.4%
Some master's degree (e.g., MA, MS, MPH, MSPH, MHA, MEd)	1223	60.9%
Education Specialist (EdS)	5	0.2%
Doctorate (e.g., PhD, EdD, JD, MD, DrPH)	338	16.9%
Total	**2008***	**100%**
Highest degree obtained that includes major emphasis on health education		
Bachelors	496	24.7%
Master's degree other than MPH or MSPH	491	24.5%
Master of Public Health	698	34.8%
Doctorate other than Public Health	171	8.5%
Doctor of Public Health	89	4.4%
Other	55	2.7%
None	8	0.4%
Total	**2008***	**100%**

*Total n varies based on participant responses

Table: 2.2

Professional Data of Survey Participants

Characteristics	n*	Percent
NCHEC Credentials		
CHES®	1584	78.8%
MCHES®	335	16.7%
No, never held either CHES® or MCHES®	80	4.0%
No, lapsed CHES® or MCHES®	12	0.6%
Total	**2011***	**100%**
Other Certifications dealing with health education/promotion		
Wellness Coach–NBC-HWP or similar certification	136	33.9%
Registered Nurse–RN	69	17.2%
Child Passenger Safety–CPS	60	15.0%
Certified in Public Health–CPH	59	14.7%
Registered Dietitian–RD	40	10.0%
Certified Diabetes Educator–CDE	20	5.0%
Certified Prevention Specialist–CPS	17	4.2%
Total	**401***	**100%**
Years of experience as Health Education Specialist		
0 to 4 years	607	30.9%
5 to 9 years	477	24.3%
10 to 14 years	284	14.4%
15 to 19 years	209	10.6%
20 to 24 years	174	8.9%
25 to 29 years	86	4.4%

Characteristics	n*	Percent
Years of experience as Health Education Specialist (continued)		
30 to 34 years	72	3.7%
35 to 39 years	47	2.4%
40+ years	10	0.5%
Total	**1966***	**100%**
Years in current position		
0 to 4 years	1321	66.1%
5 to 9 years	339	17.0%
10 to 14 years	157	7.9%
15 to 19 years	85	4.3%
20 to 24 years	52	2.6%
25 to 29 years	21	1.1%
30 to 34 years	17	0.9%
35 to 39 years	5	0.3%
40+ years	2	0.1%
Total	**1999***	**100%**
Membership in health education professional associations		
Society for Public Health Education (SOPHE)	618	30.9%
American Public Health Association–Public Health Education and Health Promotion Section (APHA-PHEHP)	401	20.1%
Eta Sigma Gamma (ESG)	219	11.0%

Continued from page 22

Characteristics	n*	Percent
Membership in health education professional associations (continued)		
American College Health Association (ACHA)	79	4.0%
American School Health Association (ASHA)	60	3.0%
Society of Health and Physical Educators (SHAPE America)	50	2.5%
American College of Sports Medicine (ACSM)	43	2.2%
American Public Health Association–School Health Education and Services Section (APHA-SHES)	38	1.9%
International Union for Health Promotion and Education (IUHPE)	17	0.9%

Characteristics	n*	Percent
Membership in health education professional associations (continued)		
American Academy of Health Behavior (AAHB)	12	0.6%
National Public Health Information Coalition (NPHIC)	6	0.3%
Society of State Leaders of Health and Physical Education	5	0.3%
Local, state, or regional affiliate of a national organization	449	22.5%
Total	**1997***	**100%**

*Total n varies based on participant responses

Participants were also asked to identify their work setting using the Bureau of Labor Statistics (BLS) categories. BLS recognizes several work settings for health educators (i.e., health education specialists) although the settings are somewhat different from those presented in Table 2.3. HESPA I 2015 and HESPA II 2020 both asked respondents about their work in terms of BLS categories so as to allow a comparison of the study population against this only nationally available data set. There was general similarity (i.e., both surveys had many respondents who worked in health care or for the government), but the BLS categories have changed over time, making precise comparisons difficult.

Generic Sub-competencies

Replicating a process used in prior studies (Doyle et al., 2012; Gilmore, et al., 2005; McKenzie, et al., 2016), Scantron employees calculated composite scores for each Sub-competency using the formula: Composite = importance + (frequency − 1). The composite score generated for each Sub-competency represented a stronger weighting for the importance of a Sub-competency to the job in relation to the frequency at which health education specialists practiced. This method of weighting resulted in the lowest scores for Sub-competencies which participants deemed both unimportant and infrequently performed as indicated by a composite score of less than 3.0.

Table: 2.3
Work Settings of Survey Participants

Setting	n*	Percent
Public Health agency • Municipal, county, or district department or agency • State department or agency • Federal department or agency • Other public health agency	461	22.9%
Health care • Hospital • Non-hospital health care facility • Health plan • Other health care	361	18.0%
Academia • Academia (college or university)	348	17.3%
Community • Health planning agency • Voluntary health agency • Non-profit health education center • Non-profit health organization • Other non-profit organization w/ occasional health initiatives • Other community	336	16.7%
Business/Worksite • Business or industry • Worksite • Health insurance • For-profit contracting agency • Organized labor • Other business/worksite	167	8.3%

Setting	n*	Percent
University and College health • University or college health services	110	5.5%
School health • Pre-K, elementary, and/or secondary school • School district • State education department • Other school health	82	4.1%
Retired • Retired but practiced in the past 12 months	14	0.7%
Other • Self-employed • Professional association • Military • Intergovernmental organizations • International/NGO • Other	132	6.6%
Total	**2011**	**100%**

Table: 2.4

Work Settings of Survey Participants Using Bureau of Labor Statistics (BLS) Categories

Setting	n*	Percent
Government	660	32.9%
Hospitals; state, local, & private	358	17.8%
Religious, grantmaking, civic, professional, & similar organizations	150	7.5%
Individual and family services	90	4.5%
Outpatient care centers	78	3.9%
Other	673	33.5%
Total	**2009**	**100%**

The HEPP defined generic Sub-competencies as those Sub-competencies performed by health education specialists regardless of practice setting. For a survey project like HESPA II 2020, which makes use of rating scales, coefficient alpha is an appropriate estimation strategy. Scantron staff computed coefficient alpha statistics for each Competency and Sub-competency as they are categorized into Areas of Responsibility. This computation was also performed for the Knowledge items as they are grouped within the ten topics. Coefficient alpha statistics can range from 0 to 1, and the closer to 1 they are, the more reliable the measure is said to be. When coefficient alpha statistics equal or exceed 0.70, the measure is considered to be sufficiently reliable for general purposes. The statistics obtained for the HESPA II 2020 Competency survey and Knowledge survey all exceeded the 0.70 threshold.

Entry- and Advanced-level Sub-competencies

One important outcome of the HESPA II 2020 study was the development of a framework to describe the practice of the health education profession. To explore if the hierarchical structure validated through the CUP, HEJA 2010 and HESPA I 2015 Models was still a useful way to delineate practice, Scantron used two research questions for the practice analysis to identify entry-level and advanced-level Competencies and Sub-competencies. Those questions are:

• What are the Areas of Responsibility, Competencies, and Sub-competencies in the practice of entry-level health education specialists?

• What are the Areas of Responsibility, Competencies, and Sub-competencies in the practice of advanced-level health education specialists?

For the purpose of the practice analysis, a Competency or Sub-competency would be included in the model if:

(a) panelists reached consensus that the statement should be included with the language given and

(b) the ratings collected in the survey were sufficient to support the statement's relevance to practice.

For the analysis of ratings, and to guide the TAG's data-based decision making, a threshold had to be established to identify which elements of the model were sufficiently valid to be retained and which should be eliminated.

In preparation for the decision making related to these questions, Scantron staff conducted a Rasch analysis, deriving a measure of endorsement for each Area of Responsibility, Competency, and Sub-competency based on the ratings collected. Scantron staff also conducted a discriminant function analysis for the ratings collected for each of these statements, based on an experience classification and an education classification. An analysis of variance (ANOVA) comparing means for experience classifications and education for each rating scale was also intended to support decision making related to these questions.

As had been done in HESPA I 2015, Scantron staff computed the mean composite for every Sub-competency. The resulting mean was then compared to the threshold that had been used in HESPA I 2015, which was 3.0. The TAG agreed that the Sub-competencies that met or exceeded this threshold were endorsed at a sufficient level for Importance and Frequency to be included in the final hierarchical model. All Sub-competency statements exceeded the threshold when the data from all respondents were considered. A follow-up comparison of composite means by practice setting showed that all Competency statements exceeded the threshold for all practice settings with the exception of the Business/Worksite practice setting where they were slightly lower than 3.0 for 13 Sub-competencies. The TAG decided to retain all of the Sub-competency statements, given that practitioners in the Business/Worksite setting account for only 7.6% of the total and the means were not far below 3.0.

A decision tree was developed and implemented to identify which elements of the model could be classified at the three levels. The decision tree provided a data-based process for making Sub-competency classifications, which in turn resulted in the classification of Competencies. This process involved the comparison of findings from two experience groups and two groups formed on the basis of respondents' highest level of education in health education. All 193 Sub-competencies in the final model were classified using the decision tree, with 114 classified as entry-level. Those classified as advanced-level were further categorized as advanced-1 level (n = 59) and advanced-2 level (n = 20) using previous classifications at this level and the expert judgment of TAG members. The advanced-1 level and advanced-2 level classifications are informative for curriculum planning and similar

purposes. Only the entry-level and advanced-level classifications pertain to the certification examinations.

The Validated Model
Through the HESPA II 2020 process, the Model of practice of health education has been updated, refined, and validated. The HESPA II 2020 Model now consists of 193 Sub-competencies organized into 35 Competencies within Eight Areas of Responsibility:

Eight Areas of Responsibility of Health Education Specialists

I.	Assessment of Needs and Capacity
II.	Planning
III.	Implementation
IV.	Evaluation and Research
V.	Advocacy
VI.	Communication
VII.	Leadership and Management
VIII.	Ethics and Professionalism

The results of the HESPA II 2020 study re-verified the three distinct levels of practice established in the CUP, HEJA 2010, and HESPA I 2015 Models, i.e., the entry-level, advanced 1-level and advanced 2-level. In addition to the Areas of Responsibilities and Competencies, the HESPA II 2020 study also identified 193 Sub-competencies. Those validated at the entry-level are required for health education specialists near the beginning of their professional development. Additional Sub-competencies were validated only for more experienced health education specialists, although in this hierarchical model in which each level provides the foundation for the next level, more experienced practitioners are still expected to be competent in the entry-level Sub-competencies. Specific numbers of Competencies and Sub-competencies for each Area of Responsibility are listed as follows:

Area of Responsibility I:
4 Competencies - 25 Sub-competencies
- 22 entry-level
- 3 advanced 1-level
- 0 advanced 2-level

Area of Responsibility II:
4 Competencies -19 Sub-competencies
- 11 entry-level
- 8 advanced 1-level
- 0 advanced 2-level

Area of Responsibility III:
3 Competencies - 16 Sub-competencies
- 15 entry-level
- 1 advanced 1-level
- 0 advanced 2-level

Area of Responsibility IV:
5 Competencies - 37 Sub-competencies
- 6 entry-level
- 16 advanced 1-level
- 15 advanced 2-level

Area of Responsibility V:
4 Competencies - 18 Sub-competencies
- 16 entry-level
- 2 advanced 1-level
- 0 advanced 2-level

Area of Responsibility VI:
6 Competencies - 26 Sub-competencies
- 24 entry-level
- 1 advanced 1-level
- 1 advanced 2-level

Area of Responsibility VII:
5 Competencies - 31 Sub-competencies
- 6 entry-level
- 23 advanced 1-level
- 2 advanced 2-level

Area of Responsibility VIII:
4 Competencies - 21 Sub-competencies
- 14 entry-level
- 5 advanced 1-level
- 2 advanced 2-level

The full resulting hierarchical model is presented with the pertinent classification in Section III of this publication.

Verified Knowledge Items

The third and final research question of HESPA II 2020 pertained to health education knowledge:
- What baseline knowledge is required to perform the Areas of Responsibility, Competencies, and Sub-competencies for health education specialists?

Thus, the HEPP developed a set of Knowledge items based on those used in the previous studies, HEJA 2010 and HESPA I 2015, and augmented with emerging areas of knowledge. A list of 149 Knowledge items, organized into 10 conceptually related topic areas was determined through the consensus of the HEPP. Those topic areas were: Health Education Profession; Theories, Techniques; Ethics; Capacity and Community Building; Systems; Research, Evaluation and Data Collection; Management, Budget, Administration and Human Resources; Communication; Advocacy; and Other.

As noted earlier, one-fifth of respondents who qualified to participate in the survey were randomly assigned to the Knowledge survey. A total of 149 Knowledge items were included on the survey. Rating scales for Importance and Frequency were identical to those on the Competency portion of the survey. The 771 responses to the Knowledge survey were analyzed using the formula identical to the one employed to compute composite scores for Competencies, that is: Composite = Importance + (Frequency − 1).

Knowledge items with a composite value of less than 3.0 received further evaluation. If the average composite value for five of the seven types of work setting community, health care, public health agency, school, worksites, academia, and university wellness) was 3.0 or more, the statement was retained. Four statements did not reach this threshold and were eliminated. The four statements removed from the listing were: a) family engagement models, b) fundraising principles, c) legislative and regulatory processes, and d) policy analysis. Of the proposed Knowledge items, 145 were validated (See section VI for the full list of verified Knowledge items.)

DISCUSSION

Validated Areas of Responsibility, Competencies, and Sub-competencies

The HESPA II 2020 Model represents the fifth time the health education profession has validated the Areas of Responsibility, Competencies, and Sub-competencies. This study resulted in an increase in the number of Areas of Responsibility from seven to eight while the number of Competencies and Sub-competencies were decreased. This decrease reflects the HEPP's attempt to combine and synthesize Competencies and Sub-competencies. This process of synthesizing information is reflected in all Areas of Responsibility; with the reduction in Competencies and Sub-competencies in the HESPA II 2020 Model aligning closely with some Competencies and Sub-competencies reflected in HESPA I 2015. The changes in Competency and Sub-competency numbers and the naming of the Areas of Responsibility from HESPA I 2015 to HESPA II 2020 are as follows:

Area of Responsibility I, Assessment of Needs and Capacity reflected a change in the number of Competencies from 7 to 4 and Sub-competencies from 33 to 25 from the HESPA I 2015 Model to HESPA II 2020 Model respectively. *Area of Responsibility II Planning*, changed from 5 to 4 Competencies, while the number

of Sub-competencies decreased significantly from 34 to 19 respectively. *Area of Responsibility III Implementation* reflected a change from 4 Competencies in HESPA I 2015 to 3 in HESPA II 2020 with the number of Sub-competencies at 29 and 16 respectively. *Area of Responsibility IV Evaluation and Research* decreased from 7 Competencies and 57 Sub-competencies in the HESPA I 2015 Model to 5 Competencies and 37 Sub-competencies in the HESPA II 2020 Model through the consolidation of Competencies as seen in the other Areas of Responsibility. *Advocacy (Area of Responsibility V) and Communications (Area of Responsibility VI)* were each validated as standalone Areas of Responsibility in HESPA II 2020. The former has 4 Competencies and 18 Sub-competencies, and the latter has 6 Competencies and 26 Sub-competencies. *Area of Responsibility VII Leadership* and Management has 5 Competencies and 31 Sub-competencies. The last *Area of Responsibility Area VIII Ethics and Professionalism* is a new responsibility, with 4 Competencies and 21 Sub-competencies.

Verified Knowledge Items

The HESPA II 2020 study is the third endeavor to validate Knowledge items within the profession. The HEJA 2010 Model represented the first attempt (Doyle et al., 2012), a summary of the foundational knowledge that health education specialists should possess to perform the Seven Areas of Responsibility effectively.

As noted by those involved in the creation of the first and second list of Knowledge items, the validated list may not be exhaustive. However, this Model includes 145 statements and 14 more than the previous list. This list of Knowledge items (see Section VI) also includes the grouping of those statements into the same 10 conceptually related topics as used in the HESPA I 2015 study. This grouping offers support to health education specialists who use the list to develop curricula or exams, plan course content, or create continuing education opportunities. As the profession moves forward, the Knowledge items should be expanded, contracted, and evolved to meet the dynamic nature of the health education profession.

Finalization of the Framework Models

After the HESPA II 2020 survey and analysis were completed, the technical report and executive summary were forwarded to the SOPHE Board of Trustees and the NCHEC Board of Commissioners for consideration and acceptance. As with HEJA 2010 and HESPA I 2015, the TAG also developed a series of recommendations to the profession on uses of the HESPA II 2020 findings and implications for teaching, research and practice. The recommendations were also presented and accepted by the NCHEC and SOPHE boards.

HESPA II 2020 was conducted using methods that have been identified in the literature on practice analysis and the accreditation requirements that pertain to certification programs in the United States, that is, the National Commission for Certifying Agencies *Standards for the Accreditation of Certification Programs* (ICE, 2016) and the ISO/IEC 17024 (2012) *Conformity assessment—General requirements for bodies operating certification of persons*. The findings of the study supported decision making about the Areas of Responsibility, Competencies, Sub-competencies, and Knowledge items. Using the hierarchical model validated by means of the HESPA II 2020 surveys will provide a strong basis for demonstrating the relationship between practice and certification examination content for the CHES® and MCHES® programs. NCHEC and the various stakeholders in its certification programs can be confident that the linkage to the current practice of health education specialists is strong. Additionally, educational programs at colleges and universities, as well as continuing education providers and others responsible for professional education in health education/promotion, can use the hierarchical model and the Knowledge items with confidence that content consistent with these models bears a strong and current relationship to actual practice in the field.

SUMMARY

The HESPA II 2020 Model validates the contemporary practice of entry- and advanced-level health education specialists. The steps illustrated in Figure 2.1 and accompanying timeline in Figure 2.2 outline the work of 37 volunteer professionals representing a diversity of health education work settings, educational backgrounds, and experience levels within the profession. In addition to the seven-member TAG, these volunteers included the 17-member HEPP and 13 subject matter experts who completed the pilot instrument. With valuable assistance from the HEPP, the TAG worked with the Scantron experts to complete 22 months of planning, execution, data analyses, and model development.

The HESPA II 2020 Model has yielded an updated, refined, and validated framework that outlines the current practice of health education specialists at three levels: entry-, advanced 1-, and advanced 2-levels. In addition, the knowledge base supporting the work of health education specialists was expanded within a conceptual structure and verified. The final framework consists of 193 Sub-competencies organized into 35 Competencies within Eight Areas of Responsibility. Of the Sub-competencies, 114 have been validated at entry-level, 59 have been validated at the advanced 1-level, and 20 have been validated at the advanced 2-level. The knowledge base needed by health education specialists has been organized into 10 conceptual topic areas, and 145 Knowledge items have been validated as being used by health education specialists.

More details about the HESPA II 2020 Model and Knowledge item list, as well as recommendations for their use, are included in subsequent sections of this publication. A comparison of the HESPA II 2020 Model with the CUP and HEJA 2010 Models is also provided in Section V.

SECTION II

Notes

Section III

HESPA II 2020 Model

The HESPA II 2020 Model (see Table 3.1 to 3.9) contains a set of Competencies and Sub-competencies used in both the entry- and advanced-level practice of health education specialists. These Competencies and Sub-competencies are generic across work settings and serve as the basis for professional preparation, credentialing, and professional development for all health education specialists. As with the CUP, HEJA 2010, and HESPA I 2015 Frameworks, it is recommended that the HESPA II 2020 entry-level Competencies and Sub-competencies be addressed in all undergraduate and graduate professional preparation programs. Master's level programs also should incorporate the advanced 1-level Competencies and Sub-competencies and doctoral programs should also incorporate the advanced 2-level Competencies.

It is possible that additional setting-specific Competencies and Sub-competencies may be needed in professional preparation and development efforts for some work settings. For example, those working in health care settings may need more preparation in the culture of health care organizations; those working in community health settings may need a working knowledge of public health policy; in some business or corporate settings, the application of worksite safety regulations may be needed; and, for those preparing to teach in schools, teaching methodologies may be needed.

The format used to present the Areas of Responsibility, Competencies and Sub-competencies is the same numbering system that was developed for and used in the HESPA I 2015 Model. This numbering system was retained for the HESPA II 2020 Model to provide a simple and consistent approach to label and use parts of the Model. Roman numerals still will be used when referring to the Eight Areas of Responsibility when the Areas stand alone, though Arabic numbers will be used as part of the numbering system for the Areas when referring to Competencies and Sub-competencies. In this numbering system, the first number refers to the Area of Responsibility, the second number refers to the Competency within that Area, and the third number refers to the Sub-competency. For example, the three digit number 1.2.3 represents the first Area of Responsibility, second Competency, and third Sub-competency.

AREA OF RESPONSIBILITY I: ASSESSMENT OF NEEDS AND CAPACITY

The Role
The first step in developing a health education program in any given setting is to gather data and information to assess the needs of the priority population. This needs assessment then becomes the foundation of the entire planning process. The needs assessment is used to determine priority programs and will assist in identifying the most appropriate interventions. Failure to conduct a thorough and comprehensive needs assessment can result in wasted time and resources. To successfully conduct a needs assessment, health education specialists collect and analyze both primary and secondary data. To assess capacity, the health education specialist must determine the resources that are present and available for use in developing programs to meet the needs of priority populations as identified via the needs assessment. Gaps in existing resources must be identified and addressed prior to initiating programs. No program should be initiated until there is sufficient capacity to be reasonably sure of success. As McKenzie, et al. (2017) have noted, "Conducting a needs assessment may be the most critical step in the planning process…" (p.90).

SECTION III

Table 3.1
Health Education Specialist Practice Analysis II 2020 Model: Overview of Areas of Responsibility and Competencies

	Area of Responsibility I: Assessment of Needs and Capacity
1.1	Plan assessment
1.2	Obtain primary data, secondary data, and other evidence-informed sources
1.3	Analyze the data to determine the health of the priority population(s) and the factors that influence health
1.4	Synthesize assessment findings to inform the planning process

	Area of Responsibility II: Planning
2.1	Engage priority populations, partners, and stakeholders for participation in the planning process
2.2	Define desired outcomes
2.3	Determine health education and promotion interventions
2.4	Develop plans and materials for implementation and evaluation

	Area of Responsibility III: Implementation
3.1	Coordinate the delivery of intervention(s) consistent with the implementation plan
3.2	Deliver health education and promotion interventions
3.3	Monitor implementation

	Area of Responsibility IV: Evaluation and Research
4.1	Design process, impact, and outcome evaluation of the intervention
4.2	Design research studies
4.3	Manage the collection and analysis of evaluation and/or research data using appropriate technology
4.4	Interpret data
4.5	Use findings

	Area of Responsibility V: Advocacy
5.1	Identify a current or emerging health issue requiring policy, systems, or environmental change
5.2	Engage coalitions and stakeholders in addressing the health issue and planning advocacy efforts
5.3	Engage in advocacy
5.4	Evaluate advocacy

	Area of Responsibility VI: Communication
6.1	Determine factors that affect communication with the identified audience(s)
6.2	Determine communication objective(s) for audience(s)
6.3	Develop message(s) using communication theories and/or models
6.4	Select methods and technologies used to deliver message(s)
6.5	Deliver the message(s) effectively using the identified media and strategies
6.6	Evaluate communication

	Area of Responsibility VII: Leadership and Management
7.1	Coordinate relationships with partners and stakeholders (e.g., individuals, teams, coalitions, and committees)
7.2	Prepare others to provide health education and promotion
7.3	Manage human resources
7.4	Manage fiduciary and material resources
7.5	Conduct strategic planning with appropriate stakeholders

	Area of Responsibility VIII: Ethics and Professionalism
8.1	Practice in accordance with established ethical principles
8.2	Serve as an authoritative resource on health education and promotion
8.3	Engage in professional development to maintain and/or enhance proficiency
8.4	Promote the health education profession to stakeholders, the public, and others

Section III: HESPA II 2020 Model

Setting: The following text is presented to describe how assessment is used in different practice settings.

Community Setting: In a community setting, health education specialists rely on many sources of primary and secondary data to determine the needs of those in the priority population. Such data can come from external sources including health planning agencies, public health departments, census reports, data sets (e.g., Behavioral Risk Factor Surveillance System and Youth Risk Behavior Surveillance System), and literature reviews. Integration of public health datasets with GIS software provides a link between a priority community and its health characteristics. Critical data are also collected internally from the proposed setting and the priority population including focus groups, town hall meetings, and interviews with community leaders and members, especially when assessing capacity. Health education specialists will assess capacity considering resources such as organizational infrastructure, staff, previous and current programming efforts, readiness, and budget when available. Data provide information about both real and perceived health needs and capacity. Depending on the types of needs identified, a well-planned health education program could address these needs if the capacity exists to do so. For example, if specific behaviors or health practices are causally linked to the incidence of major health problems, then a health education program can be planned to motivate and facilitate voluntary, desirable changes in those behaviors (e.g., develop an educational campaign for communities with high numbers of immunization avoidant parents [perceived risk/misinformation] and the outcome of a recent disease outbreak [known risks/complications], such as the measles). The needs assessment may also point to needed policy or environmental changes that the health education specialist may advocate for and support as appropriate.

School (K-12) Setting: Health education specialists in a K-12 setting rely primarily on local data to determine the needs of the youth population, although state and national data may indicate trends which can be helpful in local planning. Ideally schools will utilize the Whole School, Whole Community, Whole Child (WSCC) model, which is an expansion and update of the Coordinated School Health (CSH) approach. The WSCC model focuses its attention on the child, emphasizes a school-wide approach, and acknowledges learning, health, and the school as an important part of the local community. Data should be gathered directly from students to assess their health knowledge, attitudes, skills, and practices. The data will be used to guide instruction, school policies, and modifications in the school environment. Data should also be gathered from parents and administrators to determine potential gaps and/or barriers to health education in the school setting. Further, a community assessment should be completed to determine assets in the community that may be utilized and possible gaps in the community that should be addressed.

Health Care Setting: In the health care setting, health education specialists may be utilized to assess and review existing and/or new reports and data collected from different sources to improve health care delivery. The sources of data could include the Electronic Health Record (EHR), Electronic Medical Record (EMR), safety data such as incident reports, The Hospital Consumer Assessment of Healthcare Providers and Systems (HCAHPS), and other patient satisfaction assessment tools such as the Press-Ganey Survey. Health education specialists must be able to conduct online research and literature reviews using various medical and scientific databases including MedlinePlus, PubMed, online journals, and other core databases. For a practical example, suppose clinical staff become concerned about patients' compliance in taking their prescribed medicine and its impact on the growing number of emergency room visits. The health education specialist is given the responsibility to examine this concern and begins by conducting a needs/capacity assessment. The health education specialist may utilize gap analysis techniques to identify existing process, existing outcome(s), desired outcome(s), and document the need(s). In addition, a capacity assessment should be completed to assess and identify the stakeholders, availability of staff, aides, volunteers, funding, and other resources needed to address prescription medicine compliance and ultimately improve patient outcomes and patient experience. In another example, health education specialists may work directly with patients and/or staff to improve their health behaviors and health status. In this situation the health education specialist may use a needs assessment survey, direct individual interviewing, focus groups, and/or review the medical records of the priority population to determine health needs, and determine interest in learning opportunities, educational programs, and classes offered in a health care setting. When assessing health education needs in a clinical setting, health education specialists may assess the priority populations' knowledge, perceptions, attitudes, motivations, health literacy, health numeracy, linguistic preferences, and cultural and religious beliefs regarding their current health status. This information is specifically useful to address any potential changes that the patients and/or staff members may be considering in order to improve and/or maintain their health.

College/University Setting: In the college or university setting, health education specialists often serve as faculty and are involved in assessing student academic performance via formative and summative assessments to meet state and national certification/licensure standards, as well as to meet program accreditation requirements. For example, a review of curriculum to assess alignment with the expected roles and responsibilities of a health education specialist could identify gaps in professional preparation. To revise curricula and meet accreditation standards,

health education specialists also track students' progress in meeting the standards, assess the learning environment, and analyze any links between the two.

Worksite/Business Setting: Health education specialists may develop their own data collection strategies or work with health care professionals, specialty health and wellbeing vendors, and/or health insurance carriers to obtain and analyze aggregate data that can be used to identify the health needs of employees. For example, these analyses might include data from health risk assessments (HRAs), needs and interest surveys, health insurance claims, pharmacy data, predictive modeling tools (future risk projections), disease prevalence, disability claims, and absenteeism. Analyses of these data and other data sets would indicate priority needs for worksite programs.

College/University Health Promotion Services Setting: Health education specialists in this setting work closely with clinical practitioners and staff in health, counseling, student life, human resources, and fitness/wellness centers. They determine the individual and community health needs of students, faculty, and staff through the use of multiple strategies including, for example, focus groups, surveys, and interviews. In the assessment process, health education specialists develop avenues for obtaining information on the priority populations' knowledge, skills, perceptions, attitudes, beliefs, behaviors, learning preferences, and perceived needs in addition to health problems. In addition, available resources must be identified and needed resources must be obtained. Once data are collected, health education specialists analyze them to determine need and identify capacity, including factors that may impact the effectiveness of health education and promotion programs and interventions. These assessments form the basis for establishing priorities and recommendations for programs and interventions within the campus health promotion services setting.

Table 3.2
Health Education Specialist Practice Analysis II 2020 Model: Area of Responsibility I: Assessment of Needs and Capacity

Area of Responsibility I: Assessment of Needs and Capacity					
Entry-level Sub-competencies		Advanced 1-level Sub-competencies		Advanced 2-level Sub-competencies	
Competency 1.1 Plan assessment					
1.1.1	Define the purpose and scope of the assessment				
1.1.2	Identify priority population(s)				
1.1.3	Identify existing and available resources, policies, programs, practices, and interventions				
1.1.4	Examine the factors and determinants that influence the assessment process				
1.1.5	Recruit and/or engage priority population(s), partners, and stakeholders to participate throughout all steps in the assessment, planning, implementation, and evaluation processes				
Competency 1.2 Obtain primary data, secondary data, and other evidence-informed sources					
1.2.1	Identify primary data, secondary data, and evidence-informed resources				
		1.2.2	Establish collaborative relationships and agreements that facilitate access to data		
1.2.3	Conduct a literature review				
1.2.4	Procure secondary data				
1.2.5	Determine the validity and reliability of the secondary data				
1.2.6	Identify data gaps				
1.2.7	Determine primary data collection needs, instruments, methods, and procedures				

Area of Responsibility I: Assessment of Needs and Capacity					
Entry-level Sub-competencies		Advanced 1-level Sub-competencies		Advanced 2-level Sub-competencies	
Competency 1.2 Obtain primary data, secondary data, and other evidence-informed sources (continued)					
1.2.8	Adhere to established procedures to collect data				
		1.2.9	Develop a data analysis plan		
Competency 1.3 Analyze the data to determine the health of the priority population(s) and the factors that influence health					
1.3.1	Determine the health status of the priority population(s)				
1.3.2	Determine the knowledge, attitudes, beliefs, skills, and behaviors that impact the health and health literacy of the priority population(s)				
1.3.3	Identify the social, cultural, economic, political, and environmental factors that impact the health and/or learning processes of the priority population(s)				
1.3.4	Assess existing and available resources, policies, programs, practices, and interventions				
1.3.5	Determine the capacity (available resources, policies, programs, practices, and interventions) to improve and/or maintain health				
1.3.6	List the needs of the priority population(s)				
Competency 1.4 Synthesize assessment findings to inform the planning process					
		1.4.1	Compare findings to norms, existing data, and other information		
1.4.2	Prioritize health education and promotion needs				
1.4.3	Summarize the capacity of priority population(s) to meet the needs of priority population(s)				

Area of Responsibility I: Assessment of Needs and Capacity		
Entry-level Sub-competencies	**Advanced 1-level Sub-competencies**	**Advanced 2-level Sub-competencies**
Competency 1.4 Synthesize assessment findings to inform the planning process (continued)		
1.4.4 Develop recommendations based on findings 1.4.5 Report assessment findings		

AREA OF RESPONSIBILITY II: PLANNING

The Role

Planning begins by reviewing the health needs, problems, concerns and capacity of the priority population obtained through the assessment of needs and capacity (Responsibility I). Early in the planning process it is important to recruit interested partners and stakeholders, such as community, religious and political leaders, representatives from community organizations, resource providers and representatives of the priority population to support and help develop the program. This planning group or committee then works to develop the mission, goals and objectives as well as create or adapt intervention strategies. The intervention strategies selected must be sufficiently robust, or effective enough, to ensure the stated objectives have a reasonable chance of being met. Cottrell, et.al. (2018) call this the "Rule of Sufficiency" (p.183). Next, the planning group must locate the resources needed to implement and evaluate the program, develop a plan for delivery, and address factors that influence the implementation of the intervention. Utilizing the objectives developed during this planning phase, the health education specialist will also begin considering the process for program evaluation (Responsibility IV).

Setting: The following text is presented to describe how planning is used in different practice settings.

Community Setting: In a community setting where a needs and capacity assessment has been used to identify both a significant health problem and an opportunity to address that health problem, the role of health education specialists is to develop a comprehensive plan for implementation, evaluation, and sustainability. To begin, the health education specialist convenes representatives of relevant groups for the purpose of planning a health education/promotion program who will remain appropriately involved throughout the process. In identifying committee members, health education specialists may seek input and promote involvement from those who will affect, and be affected by, the program. Another key responsibility of health education specialists is to lead efforts to formulate goals and objectives and to adapt, or implement culturally relevant, evidence-based interventions that meet the needs of priority populations. If no appropriate programs exist, health education specialists are expected to develop evidence-informed programs and plans to evaluate preliminary impact. Health education specialists identify and assess community resources and barriers affecting the implementation of the program to achieve a successful program or intervention in the community setting.

School (K-12) Setting: National laws, local mandates, school boards and school administrators determine the requirement for providing health education in schools. Health education specialists employed in schools should select an advisory committee consisting of administrators, teachers, parents, and members of the community. The committee will identify objectives and age-appropriate curriculum, and materials/resources to meet the objectives outlined. Ideally the curriculum will follow a logical scope and sequence from K-12 and focus on the physical, mental, emotional, as well as the social and moral aspects of health for the whole child. A means to evaluate the effectiveness of the curriculum should also be designed during the planning stage. On more of a micro level, each health education specialist must plan lessons for their students on a daily basis that include learning objectives, teaching strategies, and evaluation methods.

Health Care Setting: Health education specialists in the health care setting often work collaboratively with a multidisciplinary planning team and/or a formalized advisory group to plan individual patient and population level health education programs. The team or advisory group may include physicians, nurses, advanced nurse practitioners, physician assistants, dieticians, pharmacists, social workers, members of the priority population and other stakeholders. This team utilizes the gap analysis, needs assessment and capacity data which has already been collected to design or modify educational resources, aids, and programs that can assist patients and their families to make informed decisions about their health, health care and/or lifestyle choices. The specific role of health education specialists during the planning phase is to identify program scope, to assist the team to establish mission, goals and objectives, and identify available resources that support the proposed program including any potential billable services. An evaluation plan must also be designed as part of planning. In addition, health education specialists offer advice about teaching tools, methods and strategies, and design promotion and evaluation tools needed to achieve the intended outcomes. They must be able to evaluate, develop, customize, and update patient education materials as needed. These materials may include brochures, posters, flyers, booklets, checklists, Websites, and online resources. Further, the health education specialist may be involved in developing

strategies to initiate or change policies, rules, and regulations that may impact the health of the priority population.

College/University Setting: Health education specialist faculty in a higher education setting analyze research results, current professional Competencies, certification requirements, accreditation standards, state standards and available instructional resources when planning the Health Education curriculum. Course planning is a major component of curriculum planning and health education specialists may plan courses for public health education majors as well as for the general student population. Teaching health education students how to plan programs, including the development of program goals and objectives, is vitally important. Within courses, faculty health education specialists should plan to use a variety of teaching methods, including lectures, discussions, simulations, practical experiences, and focused assignments. University health education specialists may also be given responsibility to plan class schedules, to plan budgets, and for long range program planning.

Worksite/Business Setting: Health education specialists analyze aggregate data from numerous sources that may include medical and pharmacy data, HRA data, biometric screening data, and other data sets. These data provide the basis for making a business case to key stakeholders outlining the benefits and costs of a health education program. After gaining support, health education specialists may convene an employee committee with representatives from different parts of the organization to develop a strategic plan outlining program priorities, goals and objectives, timelines, communications, incentives, and proposed budget. Health education specialists lead the team in identifying or developing evidence-based interventions and strategies to meet the needs of employees. A plan to evaluate the interventions and strategies should be developed at this point. Health education specialists also identify opportunities for new or updated policies that support employees' health and wellbeing. Examples of such policies include tobacco-free worksites, healthy vending machine and cafeteria selections, and flex time to participate in health promotion activities.

College/University Health Promotion Services Setting: Health education specialists in this setting review and utilize assessment results in collaboration with other university personnel such as practitioners in health, counseling, student life, human resources, and fitness/wellness centers. This team works together to develop program goals and objectives, as well as to select and design evidence-informed and theory-based programs and interventions that address

issues and improve health within a socioecological systems perspective. Health education specialists develop partnerships with clinical practitioners, faculty members, students, off campus agencies, and other stakeholders to integrate health education into other programs, including treatment protocols and campus wide activities. Within the planning process health education specialists place emphasis on tailoring materials, methods, and technology that appeal to student preferences and the diverse and changing populations represented on a university campus. An important component of planning is to develop an evaluation process that will be utilized to determine the effectiveness of any initiated programs.

SECTION III

Table 3.3
Health Education Specialist Practice Analysis II 2020 Model: Area of Responsibility II: Planning

Area of Responsibility II: Planning					
Entry-level Sub-competencies		Advanced 1-level Sub-competencies		Advanced 2-level Sub-competencies	
Competency 2.1 Engage priority populations, partners, and stakeholders for participation in the planning process					
2.1.1	Convene priority populations, partners, and stakeholders				
2.1.2	Facilitate collaborative efforts among priority populations, partners, and stakeholders				
2.1.3	Establish the rationale for the intervention				
Competency 2.2 Define desired outcomes					
2.2.1	Identify desired outcomes using the needs and capacity assessment				
2.2.2	Elicit input from priority populations, partners, and stakeholders regarding desired outcomes				

Area of Responsibility II: Planning					
Entry-level Sub-competencies		**Advanced 1-level Sub-competencies**		**Advanced 2-level Sub-competencies**	
Competency 2.2 Define desired outcomes (continued)					
2.2.3	Develop vision, mission, and goal statements for the intervention(s)				
2.2.4	Develop specific, measurable, achievable, realistic, and time-bound (SMART) objectives				
Competency 2.3 Determine health education and promotion interventions					
2.3.1	Select planning model(s) for health education and promotion				
		2.3.2	Create a logic model		
		2.3.3	Assess the effectiveness and alignment of existing interventions to desired outcomes		
2.3.4	Adopt, adapt, and/or develop tailored intervention(s) for priority population(s) to achieve desired outcomes				
		2.3.5	Plan for acquisition of required tools and resources		
		2.3.6	Conduct a pilot test of intervention(s)		
		2.3.7	Revise intervention(s) based on pilot feedback		
Competency 2.4 Develop plans and materials for implementation and evaluations					
		2.4.1	Develop an implementation plan inclusive of logic model, work plan, responsible parties, timeline, marketing, and communication		
2.4.2	Develop materials needed for implementation				
2.4.3	Address factors that influence implementation				
		2.4.4	Plan for evaluation and dissemination of results		
		2.4.5	Plan for sustainability		

AREA OF RESPONSIBILITY III: IMPLEMENTATION

The Role

Utilizing work accomplished in the needs/capacity assessment (Responsibility I) and in planning (Responsibility II), it is now time to implement the programs. This involves coordinating the logistics to train volunteers and staff, delivering the program, monitoring the progress, and evaluating the effectiveness and sustainability of the program. To successfully implement a program, health education specialists must have a thorough understanding of the people in the priority population: What is their current level of understanding regarding the health issue? What will it take to get the priority population to participate in a program? Do they need financial assistance or child care? What time of the day should the program be offered? What location(s) would be most convenient? and so on. For many health education specialists, implementation is one of the more enjoyable responsibilities as it may involve actually delivering the program to the priority population. It is important to note that none of the Areas of Responsibility stand alone, but are interconnected with the other Areas of Responsibility. For example, during implementation the health education specialist typically has the most contact with the public, so it is essential to act in an ethical and professional manner (Responsibility VIII). Effective communication skills (Responsibility VI) are a necessity. In most programs health education specialists will also be using population-based approaches that focus on policies, rules, regulations and laws to improve the health of priority populations. This will require advocacy skills (Responsibility V). Further leadership and management skills (Responsibility VII) are needed to actually develop and deliver a program. It is remarkable how all of the responsibilities work together and are required for a successful health education program.

Setting: The following text is presented to describe how implementation is used in different practice settings.

Community Setting: Once a health education program and plan has been designed for a priority population, health education specialists must work to identify and obtain the resources to implement the program. Information gathered from the needs and capacity assessment will inform this process. Personnel are a primary resource in implementing any such program. Health education specialists will need to train staff members and volunteers or obtain assistance from a community coalition to implement the program. Training must encompass ethics, cultural considerations, troubleshooting, and any quality assurance/fidelity processes in addition to actual delivery of the program. After launching the program, health education specialists continue to monitor progress, retain appropriate documentation, and consider various strategies for sustaining the program over time which may include transitioning program oversight to the community.

School (K-12) Setting: The health education specialist will assist youth learners in attaining, sustaining, and promoting life-long health and wellness. The K-12 curriculum should provide opportunities for the development of health literacy competencies among students and positively influence their overall well-being. The health education specialist develops age-appropriate learning objectives and activities to promote positive health behaviors. Further, the health education specialist will monitor student learning to facilitate revisions in curricula and instructional methods. This includes scaffolding on student experience and prior learning; utilizing culture-responsive scenarios and materials; incorporating arts; engaging learners in meaningful simulations and cooperative learning activities; and using life skills and value-based strategies. The teacher should also use differentiated instruction in order to reach students' various needs and abilities.

In addition, health education specialists should work with the established advisory committee to establish and implement school policies that support healthy behaviors.

Health Care Setting: Actually, implementing or oversight for implementing programs is often the responsibility of the health education specialist and the planning team. In the health care setting, health education specialists often serve as liaisons between patients and the health care team to enhance patient experience and help them understand the nature of their condition and its treatment. In addition, they may serve as outreach coordinators and provide programs in the community the health care system serves, or as program coordinators, and/or program managers and provide patient or staff education programs in the health care facilities. Thus, health education specialists in this setting might conduct patient and/or community education programs to improve patient outcomes, to support disease prevention, and to promote healthy lifestyle behaviors. They may facilitate and/or deliver programs and classes designed to address a specific health topic based on current medical and scientific evidence-based practice guidelines approved by specialists in the field. For example, health education specialists in this setting might conduct a program to support patients' weight-loss efforts on an individual level. They may also offer group classes, supported by presentations from health care providers and develop strategies to offer healthy alternatives in vending machines. Health education specialists might arrange opportunities to apply information learned through cooking classes or a grocery store tour to improve patients' ability to shop wisely and read food labels. It is important for the health education specialist to monitor the programs' processes and outcomes to make necessary changes to the program and its delivery as warranted. Evaluation data are typically collected during this phase.

College/University Setting: Health education specialists working in a higher education setting use their knowledge and skills to implement academic programs designed to prepare future health education specialists and/or promote personal and community health among the general student population. Health education specialists may also implement programs in a community, K-12 school or college setting as part of their research or community service that are designed to improve the health of the priority population. Implementation includes the use of a variety of instructional and assessment methods designed to promote higher-order thinking, knowledge acquisition, behavior change and/or the authentic application of requisite Competencies. It is of utmost importance for the health education specialist to provide culturally appropriate, relevant, and engaging learning opportunities for students or a priority population that ensure program success. Health education specialist faculty must also teach implementation skills to their students to ensure the Competencies and Sub-competencies of a health education specialist have been met.

Worksite/Business Setting: Health education specialists work with employers to offer programs and recommend policies that respond to employees' health and wellbeing needs. These programs and policies also have multiple aims to have a positive influence on employee recruitment and retention, morale, engagement, absenteeism, and/or health care costs. Health education specialists must understand the needs and interests of employees, the workplace culture, job functions, and business practices that might affect health-related behaviors. When initiating programs, it is important to monitor program fidelity and to periodically gauge how the program is being received by the priority population. Health education specialists may advocate for policies to offer healthful food choices in the company cafeteria and/or vending machines and program opportunities for physical activity, nutrition, stress management, tobacco cessation, sleep health, diabetes prevention, and others.

College/University Health Promotion Services Setting: Health education specialists in this setting work with other practitioners, stakeholders, and peer educators on campus to implement programs that address established needs utilizing a variety of evidence-informed and theory-based strategies. Health education specialists may coordinate special events, develop health initiatives, arrange for screenings by other agencies, or develop programs for priority populations within the campus community. Priority populations in this setting can include students, faculty and/or staff members. Program settings vary, and can include academic classrooms, residence halls, athletic team meeting rooms, Greek houses, and faculty/staff members gathering places. For example, health education specialists may work with residence hall staff to offer educational sessions on several topics, including safer sex, use/abuse of alcohol and other drugs, relationship violence, stress and time management, smoking cessation, nutrition, and physical activity. They may also work with individual students, faculty, and/or staff to conduct one-on-one health coaching and motivational interviewing sessions on similar topics. Beyond group and individual programming, health education specialists may work to change campus policies, such as no smoking policies or healthy food alternatives in vending machines.

Table 3.4
Health Education Specialist Practice Analysis II 2020 Model: Area of Responsibility III: Implementation

Area of Responsibility III: Implementation					
Entry-level Sub-competencies		Advanced 1-level Sub-competencies		Advanced 2-level Sub-competencies	
Competency 3.1 Coordinate the delivery of intervention(s) consistent with the implementation plan					
3.1.1	Secure implementation resources				
3.1.2	Arrange for implementation services				
3.1.3	Comply with contractual obligations	3.1.4	Establish training protocol		
3.1.5	Train staff and volunteers to ensure fidelity				
Competency 3.2 Deliver health education and promotion interventions					
3.2.1	Create an environment conducive to learning				
3.2.2	Collect baseline data				
3.2.3	Implement a marketing plan				
3.2.4	Deliver health education and promotion as designed				

Area of Responsibility III: Implementation		
Entry-level Sub-competencies	**Advanced 1-level Sub-competencies**	**Advanced 2-level Sub-competencies**
Competency 3.2 Deliver health education and promotion interventions (continued)		
3.2.5 Employ an appropriate variety of instructional methodologies		
Competency 3.3 Monitor implementation		
3.3.1 Monitor progress in accordance with the timeline		
3.3.2 Assess progress in achieving objectives		
3.3.3 Modify interventions as needed to meet individual needs		
3.3.4 Ensure plan is implemented with fidelity		
3.3.5 Monitor use of resources		
3.3.6 Evaluate the sustainability of implementation		

AREA OF RESPONSIBILITY IV: EVALUATION AND RESEARCH

The Role

The skills necessary to conduct thorough program evaluations and original health education research have much in common. Both require health education specialists to be competent in designing plans to guide their work including selecting, adapting and or creating valid and reliable data collection instruments, developing sampling plans, collecting and managing data, analyzing collected data, interpreting results, applying findings and communicating results. Evaluation is ultimately focused on determining if program objectives (Responsibility II) have been met. Evaluation must be conducted to measure the success of health education and health promotion programs. Programs not properly evaluated may be wasting valuable time, money and effort. Research is concerned with identifying new knowledge or practices that answer questions and/or test hypotheses about a health-related theory, behavior or phenomenon. Research is necessary to keep the health education profession moving forward and improving. While all health education specialists need to be competent in the basic skills of evaluation and research, much of this work, because of its complexity, is completed by those with advanced-level training and several years of work experience.

Setting: The following text is presented to describe how evaluation and research is used in different practice settings.

Community Setting: Health education specialists in a community setting must understand and interpret evaluation and research findings for use in their work. Their work may include the use of epidemiological principles to explain disease outbreaks or define high-risk neighborhoods within communities that require special program emphasis. Their work may also include evaluating policies, systems and environmental changes in the community. Health education specialists must master research principles and language to discuss any topic important to the community, such as unintentional injuries, an outbreak of measles or food poisoning, or sexually transmitted infections. They also must understand the importance of conducting and interpreting the results of sound evaluations. Evaluations provide necessary evidence to support programs when reviewed by local or state governments. In general, health education specialists working at the entry-level may be involved in data collection for both research and evaluations, as well as interpreting the results of each of these processes. Those health education specialists working at an advanced-level of practice are responsible for planning and implementing the research and evaluation processes. It is also expected that evaluation and research findings be shared with the profession so that health education specialists may learn from each other's work and the overall performance of the profession be improved.

School (K-12) Setting: Health education specialists will routinely evaluate the attainment of student learning objectives for each lesson at each grade level and assist in the data collection to assess student health knowledge, attitudes, and behaviors. Combined with current research of literature, health education specialists identify, select, and implement effective curriculum and teaching methods to enhance health education in schools. Accountability is essential to ensure that students are receiving adequate, culturally sensitive, and effective health instruction.

Health Care Setting: Research is increasingly important in addressing health issues, chronic disease conditions and the reduction of health risk behaviors for primary prevention. Health education specialists employed in health care settings, may be involved as a member of a research team that conducts research studies to improve the quality of health and patient care. They must be able to understand research studies, answer questions from patients and their families/caregivers about the studies and interpret research findings for patients and their families. Health education specialists must be able to identify and analyze medically recommended best practices (i.e., U.S. Preventative Task Force) and incorporate them into their programs. In addition, they may collect or assist in the collection of primary, secondary, and/or tertiary data from their priority population. Health education specialists need skills to conduct summative and formative evaluation. Evaluation data is needed to support existing programs, demonstrate the need to modify existing programs, or to support future programs and program growth. Thus, health education specialists must be able to design evaluation plans to assess the effectiveness of programs and specifically the programs' ability to meet stated goals and objectives.

College/University Setting: Health education specialists in this setting are responsible for evaluating student learning as well as teaching course and program effectiveness. In some cases, college/university faculty members have responsibilities in teaching research and evaluation skills to students. Program evaluation responsibilities may also extend to community health education and promotion programs. Depending on their faculty role and university priorities, college/university health education specialists have varying levels of research responsibilities. Research responsibilities may center on health behavior research or profession-related research. Health education specialist faculty are often expected to disseminate the findings of their research and evaluation efforts through peer-reviewed publications and presentations that provide direction for future practice and research. Evaluation and research related grant-writing may be another expectation. These efforts contribute to the scientific body of knowledge encompassing health behavior, disease prevention, and risk reduction strategies, as well as to the profession of health education.

Worksite/Business Setting: Health education specialists in this setting need both qualitative and quantitative evaluation skills to demonstrate the efficacy of health education and health promotion programs and the contributions of such programs to employee satisfaction, morale, productivity, engagement, health care costs, and to organizational goals. Health education specialists may be asked to assist in monitoring the work environment for safety compliance and injury reduction. Additionally, using evaluative research, health education specialists may be able to help determine quality ("value-on-investment") and cost-effectiveness ("return-on-investment") of various internal programs and services and external vendor programs.

College/University Health Promotion Services Setting: Health education specialists in this setting face many of the same issues as those in the business/industry and health care settings. These health education specialists need skills in all facets of evaluation, must be able to understand and interpret research findings for use in practice, and may also need to conduct research. Evaluation research skills are necessary to determine the efficacy and cost-effectiveness of programs and interventions for students, staff members, and faculty members. Health education specialists are expected to communicate findings and solicit feedback from stakeholders. Findings and feedback are incorporated into improvement and sustainability of current and new programs and interventions, as well as advocacy and strategic planning processes. Successful and even unsuccessful program efforts should be shared in the literature so that others may learn from them and ultimately improve their efforts.

Table 3.5
Health Education Specialist Practice Analysis II 2020 Model: Area of Responsibility IV: Evaluation and Research

Area of Responsibility IV: Evaluation and Research					
Entry-level Sub-competencies		**Advanced 1-level Sub-competencies**		**Advanced 2-level Sub-competencies**	
Competency 4.1 Design process, impact, and outcome evaluation of the intervention					
		4.1.1	Align the evaluation plan with the intervention goals and objectives		
4.1.2	Comply with institutional requirements for evaluation				
		4.1.3	Use a logic model and/or theory for evaluations		
		4.1.4	Assess capacity to conduct evaluation		

Area of Responsibility IV: Evaluation and Research					
Entry-level Sub-competencies		**Advanced 1-level Sub-competencies**		**Advanced 2-level Sub-competencies**	
Competency 4.1 Design process, impact, and outcome evaluation of the intervention (continued)					
		4.1.5	Select an evaluation design model and the types of data to be collected		
		4.1.6	Develop a sampling plan and procedures for data collection, management, and security		
		4.1.7	Select quantitative and qualitative tools consistent with assumptions and data requirements		
4.1.8	Adopt or modify existing instruments for collecting data				
		4.1.9	Develop instruments for collecting data		
		4.1.10	Implement a pilot test to refine data collection instruments and procedures		
Competency 4.2 Design research studies					
				4.2.1	Determine purpose, hypotheses, and questions
		4.2.2	Comply with institutional and/or IRB requirements for research		
		4.2.3	Use a logic model and/or theory for research		
				4.2.4	Assess capacity to conduct research
		4.2.5	Select a research design model and the types of data to be collected		
		4.2.6	Develop a sampling plan and procedures for data collection, management, and security		

SECTION III

Area of Responsibility IV: Evaluation and Research					
Entry-level Sub-competencies		**Advanced 1-level Sub-competencies**		**Advanced 2-level Sub-competencies**	
Competency 4.2 Design research studies (continued)					
		4.2.7	Select quantitative and qualitative tools consistent with assumptions and data requirements		
				4.2.8	Adopt, adapt, and/or develop instruments for collecting data
				4.2.9	Implement a pilot test to refine and validate data collection instruments and procedures
Competency 4.3 Manage the collection and analysis of evaluation and/or research data using appropriate technology					
				4.3.1	Train data collectors
4.3.2	Implement data collection procedures				
4.3.3	Use appropriate modalities to collect and manage data				
				4.3.4	Monitor data collection procedures
4.3.5	Prepare data for analysis				
				4.3.6	Analyze data
Competency 4.4 Interpret data					
				4.4.1	Explain how findings address the questions and/or hypotheses
		4.4.2	Compare findings to other evaluations or studies		
4.4.3	Identify limitations and delimitations of findings				
				4.4.4	Draw conclusions based on findings
				4.4.5	Identify implications for practice
				4.4.6	Synthesize findings

Area of Responsibility IV: Evaluation and Research					
Entry-level Sub-competencies		**Advanced 1-level Sub-Ccmpetencies**		**Advanced 2-level Sub-competencies**	
Competency 4.4 Interpret data (continued)					
				4.4.7	Develop recommendations based on findings
				4.4.8	Evaluate feasibility of implementing recommendations
Competency 4.5 Use findings					
		4.5.1	Communicate findings by preparing reports and presentations, and by other means		
				4.5.2	Disseminate findings
				4.5.3	Identify recommendations for quality improvement
		4.5.4	Translate findings into practice and interventions		

AREA OF RESPONSIBILITY V: ADVOCACY

The Role

Health education specialists are expected to advocate for and support initiatives that promote the health of priority populations. This means they should initiate and promote legislation, laws, rules, policies and procedures that are designed to enhance health. Whether it be federal health care legislation, a state law to require motor cycle helmets, a league rule mandating mouth guards in youth basketball, or corporate policy to restrict smoking in common areas, health education specialists should have the skills to initiate and promote such initiatives. Further, health education specialists should advocate for their profession, health education certification, and accreditation of professional preparation programs. They need to educate potential employers about the benefits of hiring professionally trained, degreed and certified health education specialists. It is important that health education specialists talk to legislators, decision makers, personnel directors, allied health workers, co-workers, family and friends about the value of health education and health promotion.

Setting: The following text is presented to describe how advocacy is used in different practice settings.

Community Setting: Health education specialists act as advocates for community health needs using sound evidence and ethical principles. They may advocate for policies, laws, rules and/or regulations that promote the health of the priority population. For example, health education specialists may support, encourage or lobby the local government to use funds to develop bicycle paths or for a youth sports program to create a policy that requires all participants to wear mouth guards. Health education specialists also advocate for their own agency/

department and for the health education profession as a whole. Advocacy can take place as part of one's employment or as the civic responsibility of a private citizen.

School (K-12) Setting: In the K-12 setting, health education specialists may promote the WSCC model, which emphasizes the relationship between educational attainment and health by putting the child at the center of a system designed to support both health and education. Health education specialists may provide expert assistance to administrators in examining state and local mandates and recommending placement of health education programs in the overall curriculum scope and sequence plan. The K-12 health education specialist must be prepared to advocate for the school's health education program as well as laws, policies, rules and regulations that support youth health. The development of health councils or student health ambassador groups should also be encouraged to assist the health education specialist in advocacy efforts.

Health Care Setting: In the health care setting, the health education specialist must advocate for the health of patients and their families. In a patient-centered health care system this could involve promoting patient engagement with health care professionals, including patients in creating and developing patient education programs and materials, or advocating for organizational policy, rule or system changes that may improve the patient experience and ultimately patient health. Like health education specialists in other settings, health education specialists in the health care setting need to advocate for the health education profession and the hiring of certified health education specialists (CHES®). This may involve educating allied health professionals, staff and patients about the specific skills of a health education specialist. For example, the health education specialist may advocate for health education specialists to be given the responsibility to complete Medicare's Annual Wellness

Visit in the clinical setting per the recommendations of the Centers for Medicare and Medicaid Services.

College/University Setting: Health education specialists in the college/university setting may be charged with being advocates for health education programs at the campus level or for the health education profession at the campus, state, national or global level. In addition, the health education specialist in the college/university setting may also engage in advocacy for public health actions such as policy change or legislative action. These advocacy situations may be intended to influence campus colleagues and administrators, community members, decision-makers, and other stakeholders. Interaction with these individuals may take place in "one on one," small group or large group situations. The actions may occur in formal or informal settings, and may be planned or incidental (i.e., "the elevator speech"). Advocacy actions may also require the development of advocacy informational materials or the use of traditional or social media.

Beyond engaging in advocacy, the health education specialist working in a professional preparation program may have responsibilities in preparing prospective health education specialists in the planning, implementation and evaluation of advocacy efforts.

Worksite/Business Setting: Health education specialists may act as advocates for health education and health promotion with other functional units within the worksite including occupational health, safety, work/life, employee assistance, benefits, and other business units and functions. Health education specialists identify, organize, and advocate for resources needed for the implementation, continuation, and evaluation of programs. Health education specialists may also advocate for new policies and/or for changes to existing policies related to health and wellbeing, e.g., tobacco-free policies. They also identify data and present to key stakeholders to ensure that activities match the stated goals, objectives, outcomes, and budget. These metrics may be called key performance indicators (KPI). This often supports health education specialists' future advocacy for additional resources to modify and expand their programs. Health education specialists also need to advocate for their profession and support professional initiatives that will further the profession such as certifications and accreditations.

College/University Health Promotion Services Setting: Health education specialists in this setting advocate for support and acceptance of health education and promotion services, programs, and resources for the campus community and its members. They also advocate for policies that support health and well-being, and systems changes that ensure efficacy of health promotion services from a socioecological perspective. Health education specialists in this setting need to stay apprised of local, state, and national health issues, proposed laws/regulations, and opportunities that may impact the campus community's health. Another important advocacy role is to promote the health education profession and seek opportunities to showcase the health education specialist's important role on campus.

Table 3.6
Health Education Specialist Practice Analysis II 2020 Model: Area of Responsibility V: Advocacy

Area of Responsibility V: Advocacy					
Entry-level Sub-competencies		**Advanced 1-level Sub-competencies**		**Advanced 2-level Sub-competencies**	
Competency 5.1 Identify a current or emerging health issue requiring policy, systems, or environmental change					
5.1.1	Examine the determinants of health and their underlying causes (e.g., poverty, trauma, and population-based discrimination) related to identified health issues				
5.1.2	Examine evidence-informed findings related to identified health issues and desired changes				
5.1.3	Identify factors that facilitate and/or hinder advocacy efforts (e.g., amount of evidence to prove the issue, potential for partnerships, political readiness, organizational experience or risk, and feasibility of success)				
5.1.4	Write specific, measurable, achievable, realistic, and time-bound (SMART) advocacy objective(s)				

SECTION III

Area of Responsibility V: Advocacy					
Entry-level Sub-competencies		**Advanced 1-level Sub-competencies**		**Advanced 2-level Sub-competencies**	
Competency 5.1 Identify a current or emerging health issue requiring policy, systems, or environmental change (continued)					
5.1.5	Identify existing coalition(s) or stakeholders that can be engaged in advocacy efforts				
Competency 5.2 Engage coalitions and stakeholders in addressing the health issue and planning advocacy efforts					
5.2.1	Identify existing coalitions and stakeholders that favor and oppose the proposed policy, system, or environmental change and their reasons				
5.2.2	Identify factors that influence decision-makers (e.g., societal and cultural norms, financial considerations, upcoming elections, and voting record)				
		5.2.3	Create formal and/or informal alliances, task forces, and coalitions to address the proposed change		
5.2.4	Educate stakeholders on the health issue and the proposed policy, system, or environmental change				
5.2.5	Identify available resources and gaps (e.g., financial, personnel, information, and data)				
5.2.6	Identify organizational policies and procedures and federal, state, and local laws that pertain to the advocacy efforts				
5.2.7	Develop persuasive messages and materials (e.g., briefs, resolutions, and fact sheets) to communicate the policy, system, or environmental change				

Area of Responsibility V: Advocacy				
Entry-level Sub-competencies		Advanced 1-level Sub-competencies		Advanced 2-level Sub-competencies
Competency 5.2 Engage coalitions and stakeholders in addressing the health issue and planning advocacy efforts (continued)				
5.2.8	Specify strategies, a timeline, and roles and responsibilities to address the proposed policy, system, or environmental change (e.g., develop ongoing relationships with decision makers and stakeholders, use social media, register others to vote, and seek political appointment)			
Competency 5.3 Engage in advocacy				
5.3.1	Use media to conduct advocacy (e.g., social media, press releases, public service announcements, and op-eds)			
5.3.2	Use traditional, social, and emerging technologies and methods to mobilize support for policy, system, or environmental change			
		5.3.3	Sustain coalitions and stake-holder relationships to achieve and maintain policy, system, or environmental change	
Competency 5.4 Evaluate advocacy				
5.4.1	Conduct process, impact, and outcome evaluation of advocacy efforts			
5.4.2	Use the results of the evaluation to inform next steps			

SECTION III

AREA OF RESPONSIBILITY VI: COMMUNICATION

The Role

Communication is fundamental to all of the other Seven Responsibilities associated with being a health education specialist. Health education specialists must interact with a variety of people from various backgrounds including other health professionals, consumers, students, employers, employees, patients, and fellow health education specialists. One must be able to effectively communicate in both oral and written forms to establish and maintain successful health education programs. Whether through individual, small group, social media or mass communication strategies, health education specialists use their professional training to create, tailor, pilot test, deliver and evaluate communication messages. The ability to communicate effectively provides health education specialists with the foundation to advocate (Responsibility V) for health issues and the health education profession.

Setting: The following text is presented to describe how communication is used in different practice settings.

Community Setting: Communication is needed in nearly every aspect of a health education specialist's work within the community setting. In a community setting, health education specialists assist in developing health communication campaigns designed to bring about behavioral change among priority audiences and influence health policy issues at the local, state, and national levels. Health education specialists develop communication messages to be delivered through a variety of channels and utilize program materials developed in the language of and at appropriate reading levels of the priority population. This requires strong written and verbal skills including public speaking and the ability to identify/incorporate those communication channels used by priority populations. Competency in traditional methods of communication (i.e., radio, television, newspapers,

posters, pamphlets) and social media platforms (i.e., Twitter, Facebook, Instagram) as well as newsfeeds, webinars, and other new/emerging media platforms is especially important. Health education specialists might be asked to serve on various community-wide coalitions to help identify and implement communication strategies to improve health. Those health education specialists practicing at an advanced level may serve as communication advisors or consultants for a variety of community organizations.

School (K-12) Setting: The health education specialist must interact and communicate with a broad range of individuals including but not limited to students, parents, fellow teachers, administrators, advisory boards and the community at large. Effective communication is essential to the work of a school health education specialist. Evidence of successful implementation of the health education program should be communicated and celebrated throughout the school and community. This may involve the use of traditional communication channels such as newspapers, TV and radio as well as electronic media such as e-mail, Websites, and social media. Open forums or discussion boards should be conducted to allow for input from interested stakeholders.

Health Care Setting: In health care settings, health education specialists may serve as navigators and/or consultants assisting patients, families, caregivers, and health care providers to find evidence-based health information from reliable sources. They must have core communication skills, show empathy, be reflective listeners, and practice teach-back as they respond to patients' specific needs. They must have strong verbal and written communication skills and utilize those skills when disseminating information to patients, their families, caregivers, staff, stakeholders, and the public. When delivering health education messages and/or programs, they must be skilled in communicating scientific and medical information in an understandable format based on the learners' health literacy

Section III: HESPA II 2020 Model

and health numeracy levels. Health education specialists must be leaders and foster an inclusive workplace that promotes an environment of respect and trust through open and clear communication with all stakeholders. For a specific example, the health education specialist in the health care setting may be responsible for developing a patient-focused diabetes education communication platform for an outpatient primary care office. Upon approval, the health education specialist will then deliver the diabetes materials to the patients in multiple forms such as telephone calls, patient health portals, webinars, or via in-person sessions. As the health messages are delivered, the health education specialist evaluates the campaign to determine its effectiveness.

College/University Setting: Health education specialists in this setting communicate formally and informally with students, campus and professional colleagues, administrators and other stakeholders. The communication can occur in an instructional setting, as a member of a committee or specially designated group, at a professional conference, a public meeting or other venues. The purpose of the communication might be instructional, informational, to provide feedback or input, or for advocacy. This communication might be provided in-person, online, via e-mail, or through traditional or social media. Health education specialists working in professional preparation programs may also have responsibility for preparing prospective health education specialists to utilize communication skills. Health education specialists in a college/university setting use communication skills to disseminate evidence-based best practices and approaches for health education and health promotion. A health education specialist in this setting will use written communication to publish scholarly papers, informational papers and health education materials based on current research. Persuasive communication techniques are used by health education specialists to secure funding for grant proposals, to encourage healthy behaviors in priority populations, and to persuade decision makers

to adopt policies, laws, rules, and/or regulations to support health.

Worksite/Business Setting: Health education specialists identify and communicate unmet employee needs (e.g., insufficient opportunity for physical activity) to management and key internal stakeholders. Using their background in behavioral and biological sciences, they interpret the problem for management and articulate effective ways of addressing the problem, such as offering a program or screening or changing organizational policy. In doing so they must understand management concerns and communicate ways in which a specific health education program or policy might benefit both the organization and employees. In addition, health education specialists develop communication strategies and messages to be delivered to priority populations through a variety of channels and program materials in the style and frequency that matches the culture of the organization and supports the organization's mission, vision, values, and business practices. In this capacity health education specialists need to communicate with a variety of people (top management to hourly workers) in a variety of ways (oral, written, social media, newsletters, posters, etc.). This work may be done in conjunction with internal and/or external communications and marketing specialists.

College/University Health Promotion Services Setting: Health education specialists in this setting utilize a variety of communication strategies and channels to develop and deliver messages to priority populations, colleagues, partners, stakeholders, and administration. Communication skills are critical in assessment, program and intervention planning, marketing, implementation, and evaluation, as well as advocacy, leadership, and management. Strategies and channels used are situation specific, tailored to the audience and often include social media and digital communication for programs, interventions, and marketing with priority populations. Traditional print (e.g., posters and bulletin boards), electronic communications (e-mail, conference calls, webinars), and face-to-face communication (e.g., motivational interviewing and presentations) are also requisite skills. Health education specialists must use professional written and oral strategies when communicating with partners, stakeholders and administration. Effective communication is essential when gaining support for programs and interventions, sharing evaluation results, and advocating for resources, policies, and system changes on campus.

Table 3.7
Health Education Specialist Practice Analysis II 2020 Model: Area of Responsibility VI: Communication

Area of Responsibility VI: Communication					
Entry-level Sub-competencies		Advanced 1-level Sub-competencies		Advanced 2-level Sub-competencies	
Competency 6.1 Determine factors that affect communication with the identified audience(s)					
6.1.1	Segment the audience(s) to be addressed, as needed				
6.1.2	Identify the assets, needs, and characteristics of the audience(s) that affect communication and message design (e.g., literacy levels, language, culture, and cognitive and perceptual abilities)				
6.1.3	Identify communication channels (e.g., social media and mass media) available to and used by the audience(s)				
6.1.4	Identify environmental and other factors that affect communication (e.g., resources and the availability of Internet access)				
Competency 6.2 Determine communication objective(s) for audience(s)					
6.2.1	Describe the intended outcome of the communication (e.g., raise awareness, advocacy, behavioral change, and risk communication)				
6.2.2	Write specific, measurable, achievable, realistic, and time-bound (SMART) communication objective(s)				

Area of Responsibility VI: Communication

Entry-level Sub-competencies		Advanced 1-level Sub-competencies		Advanced 2-level Sub-competencies	
Competency 6.2 Determine communication objective(s) for audience(s) (continued from 56)					
6.2.3	Identify factors that facilitate and/or hinder the intended outcome of the communication				
Competency 6.3 Develop message(s) using communication theories and/or models					
6.3.1	Use communications theory to develop or select communication message(s)				
6.3.2	Develop persuasive communications (e.g., storytelling and program rationale)				
6.3.3	Tailor message(s) for the audience(s)				
6.3.4	Employ media literacy skills (e.g., identifying credible sources and balancing multiple viewpoints)				
Competency 6.4 Select methods and technologies used to deliver message(s)					
6.4.1	Differentiate the strengths and weaknesses of various communication channels and technologies (e.g., mass media, community mobilization, counseling, peer communication, information/digital technology, and apps)				
6.4.2	Select communication channels and current and emerging technologies that are most appropriate for the audience(s) and message(s)				
6.4.3	Develop communication aids, materials, or tools using appropriate multimedia (e.g., infographics, presentation software, brochures, and posters)				

Area of Responsibility VI: Communication				
Entry-level Sub-competencies		**Advanced 1-level Sub-competencies**	**Advanced 2-level Sub-competencies**	
Competency 6.4 Select methods and technologies used to deliver message(s) (continued)				
6.4.4	Assess the suitability of new and/or existing communication aids, materials, or tools for audience(s) (e.g., the CDC Clear Communication Index and the Suitability of Assessment Materials [SAM])			
6.4.5	Pilot test message(s) and communication aids, materials, or tools			
6.4.6	Revise communication aids, materials, or tools based on pilot results			
Competency 6.5 Deliver the message(s) effectively using the identified media and strategies				
6.5.1	Deliver presentation(s) tailored to the audience(s)			
6.5.2	Use public speaking skills			
6.5.3	Use facilitation skills with large and/or small groups			
6.5.4	Use current and emerging communication tools and trends (e.g., social media)			
6.5.5	Deliver oral and written communication that aligns with professional standards of grammar, punctuation, and style			
6.5.6	Use digital media to engage audience(s) (e.g., social media management tools and platforms)			
Competency 6.6 Evaluate communication				
6.6.1	Conduct process and impact evaluations of communications			

SECTION III

Area of Responsibility VI: Communication					
Entry-level Sub-competencies		Advanced 1-level Sub-competencies		Advanced 2-level Sub-competencies	
Competency 6.6 Evaluate communication (continued)					
				6.6.2	Conduct outcome evaluations of communications
		6.6.3	Assess reach and dose of communication using tools (e.g., data mining software, social media analytics, and Website analytics)		

AREA OF RESPONSIBILITY VII: LEADERSHIP AND MANAGEMENT

The Role

A great deal of leadership, administration, management and coordination is needed to bring a health education/promotion program to fruition. Depending on the specific work setting, some entry-level health education specialists may be called upon to lead and manage programs, but most often these are the responsibilities of health education specialists at more advanced-levels of practice. It takes good leadership and management skills to recruit partners and stakeholders who will participate in the program, but more importantly to assess their capacity and involve them in the process in meaningful ways. The effective health education specialist must be able to manage human resources and fiscal resources as well as physical resources. A good leader/manager establishes a long-range vision for the program and can work with others to develop, implement and evaluate a strategic plan. Leadership skills are not only needed in health education program development, but also within the profession. It is important that good leaders step forward to chair committees and accept positions as officers and board members. There are many health organizations, foundations, and state and national professional associations that need good leadership.

Setting: The following text is presented to describe how Leadership and Management is used in different practice settings.

Community Setting: Health education specialists in a community setting, especially those working at an advanced-level, may be responsible for managing and administering health education/promotion programs and/or organizations. Such work includes gaining acceptance for programs, utilizing evidence-based approaches, and managing the financial, technological, and human resources associated with programs. These tasks require health education specialists to create and monitor a program budget, hire and evaluate personnel, and work with both internal and external partners, as well as stakeholders, to ensure a program's success. In addition, health education specialists are responsible for managing the relationships with program partners and other stakeholders. This includes accepting cultural differences, utilizing conflict resolution skills, and ensuring that dissenting opinions are heard. In addition, health education specialists use their leadership and management skills to influence policy and advocate for positive health practices.

School (K-12) Setting: Health education specialists in K-12 schools may serve as program managers or team leaders to promote health education in their school and throughout the school district. They may have a leadership role in developing content to be addressed at each grade level in the curriculum, supervise instruction and measure learning outcomes. Health education specialists may also manage budgetary issues for the school health program and work with school leaders/stakeholders to obtain acceptance and support for health education.

Health Care Settings: Health education specialists who are employed in health care settings may hold managerial and/or leadership positions. Usually these are health education specialists who hold advanced degrees and/or have significant experience in the field. In these roles, they supervise staff and volunteers and manage professional development and continuing education programs for staff and volunteers. In addition, they may plan and implement programs that contribute to institutional maintenance of accreditation and/or compliance with government regulations. In addition, they must provide guidance and technical assistance to staff, volunteers, and health care partners. To be effective leaders, they must understand and practice ethical leadership and encourage an ethical environment and a fair and inclusive culture that promotes integrity, accountability, equality, and respect. Thus, it is essential for health education specialists at this level to have the ability to facilitate and sustain partnerships and collaborations with a variety of medical and allied health professionals, aides, volunteers, patients, families, and stakeholders in their particular health care settings. They also might participate in interdisciplinary efforts to establish advisory and consultation services to stakeholders. Health education specialists serving as managers and leaders are well positioned to ensure cultural sensitivity, diversity and inclusion by engaging a diverse group of stakeholders in every stage of program planning.

College/University Setting: Health education specialists in the college/university setting may be involved in a variety of administrative responsibilities, including coordinating professional preparation programs and chairing academic departments. In this role, health education specialists must provide program leadership, develop and/or manage program budgets, hire and supervise faculty members and staff, and be responsible for the annual evaluations of those employed in the department. They also must align their professional preparation program goals with the goals and mission of the school/college and university. In addition, health education specialists may coordinate and supervise student internships, provide leadership in course and program development and student organizations, and chair or facilitate committees and task forces. In this setting, health education specialists might be responsible for teaching competencies related to leadership and management to health education students.

Worksite/Business Setting: Health education specialists may lead or be part of a team for health education and health promotion efforts. Health education specialists may hire, supervise, provide support, and/or evaluate the performance of staff, contracted staff, vendors, and/or "wellness champion" volunteers who deliver programs virtually and/or at the worksite. Health education specialists in this setting may take the lead to develop and advocate for annual budgets and other resources that support the planning, implementation, and evaluation of worksite programs and services and policy initiatives.

College/University Health Promotion Services Setting: Health education specialists in this setting serve as leaders to provide health education and promotion services, programs, and resources for the campus community and its members. In this role they manage resources associated with programs and interventions and must demonstrate leadership through strategic planning, organizational change, and daily operations

Section III: HESPA II 2020 Model

associated with health promotion services on campus. This includes utilizing management skills such as hiring, training, evaluating, and retaining professional and student staff, developing stakeholder and partner relationships, and securing and managing financial, technological, and other resources.

Table 3.8
Health Education Specialist Practice Analysis II 2020 Model: Area of Responsibility VII: Leadership and Management

Area of Responsibility VII: Leadership and Management		
Entry-level Sub-competencies	**Advanced 1-level Sub-competencies**	**Advanced 2-level Sub-competencies**
Competency 7.1 Coordinate relationships with partners and stakeholders (e.g., individuals, teams, coalitions, and committees)		
7.1.1 Identify potential partners and stakeholders		
7.1.2 Assess the capacity of potential partners and stakeholders		
7.1.3 Involve partners and stakeholders throughout the health education and promotion process in meaningful and sustainable ways		
	7.1.4 Execute formal and informal agreements with partners and stakeholders	
7.1.5 Evaluate relationships with partners and stakeholders on an ongoing basis to make appropriate modifications		
Competency 7.2 Prepare others to provide health education and promotion		
7.2.1 Develop culturally responsive content		
7.2.2 Recruit individuals needed in implementation		
	7.2.3 Assess training needs	
	7.2.4 Plan training, including technical assistance and support	

Area of Responsibility VII: Leadership and Management		
Entry-level Sub-competencies	**Advanced 1-level Sub-competencies**	**Advanced 2-level Sub-competencies**
Competency 7.2 Prepare others to provide health education and promotion (continued)		
	7.2.5 Implement training	
	7.2.6 Evaluate training as appropriate throughout the process	
Competency 7.3 Manage human resources		
	7.3.1 Facilitate understanding and sensitivity for various cultures, values, and traditions	
	7.3.2 Facilitate positive organizational culture and climate	
	7.3.3 Develop job descriptions to meet staffing needs	
	7.3.4 Recruit qualified staff (including paraprofessionals) and volunteers	
	7.3.5 Evaluate performance of staff and volunteers formally and informally	
	7.3.6 Provide professional development and training for staff and volunteers	
	7.3.7 Facilitate the engagement and retention of staff and volunteers	
	7.3.8 Apply team building and conflict resolution techniques as appropriate	
Competency 7.4 Manage fiduciary and material resources		
	7.4.1 Evaluate internal and external financial needs and funding sources	
	7.4.2 Develop financial budgets and plans	

SECTION III

Area of Responsibility VII: Leadership and Management					
Entry-level Sub-competencies		Advanced 1-level Sub-competencies		Advanced 2-level Sub-competencies	
Competency 7.4 Manage fiduciary and material resources (continued)					
		7.4.3	Monitor budget performance		
				7.4.4	Justify value of health education and promotion using economic (e.g., cost-benefit, return-on-investment, and value-on-investment) and/or other analyses
		7.4.5	Write grants and funding proposals		
				7.4.6	Conduct reviews of funding and grant proposals
		7.4.7	Monitor performance and/or compliance of funding recipients		
		7.4.8	Maintain up-to-date technology infrastructure		
		7.4.9	Manage current and future facilities and resources (e.g., space and equipment)		
Competency 7.5 Conduct strategic planning with appropriate stakeholders					
		7.5.1	Facilitate the development of strategic and/or improvement plans using systems thinking to promote the mission, vision, and goal statements for health education and promotion		
		7.5.2	Gain organizational acceptance for strategic and/or improvement plans		
		7.5.3	Implement the strategic plan, incorporating status updates and making refinements as appropriate		

AREA OF RESPONSIBILITY VIII: ETHICS AND PROFESSIONALISM

The Role

Ethics refers to the moral principles generally accepted as the proper way to conduct oneself while working as a health education specialist. There is an official Code of Ethics for the Health Education Profession (Coalition of National Health Education Organizations, 2011; Cottrell, et.al., 2018). Professionalism relates to the accepted conduct, aims or qualities that characterize someone working in the health education profession. Examples of professionalism include practicing in accord with accepted standards, participating in continuing education, belonging to professional associations, serving on committees, attending conferences and providing leadership to the profession. Ethical behavior and professionalism are expected when assessing needs, planning programs, implementing programs, managing programs, evaluating programs and conducting research. Acting in an ethical and professional manner is always expected of health education specialists and doing so helps establish one's reputation within the community and profession. It can take years to build one's reputation within the profession, but one unethical action or unprofessional interaction can destroy that reputation.

Setting: The following text is presented to describe how ethics and professionalism is used in different practice settings.

Community Setting: Health education specialists must follow the Code of Ethics for the Health Education Profession which defines ethical behavior within the profession. In a community setting, health education specialists work to promote equitable partnerships with communities to address issues of health and maintain professional partnerships with other community stakeholders in order to effectively serve the community. This includes practicing cultural humility and treating colleagues, community partners, and priority populations with dignity at all times. Health education specialists working with numerous entities such as public health departments, community-based organizations, local voluntary health organizations, churches, civic organizations, neighborhood associations, and other nonprofits must maintain the highest of ethical and professional standards. Individual as well as agency reputations are based on ethical behavior. Health education specialists are also responsible for continual professional growth and development to remain up to date on current research, health trends, and emerging technology in order to better serve their priority populations. Professional association membership is important to stay up to date, network with other health education professionals and demonstrate commitment to the profession.

School (K-12) Setting: According to the Code of Ethics for the Health Education Profression, "The health education profession is dedicated to excellence in the practice of promoting individual, family, group, organizational and community health" (CNHEO, 2011, p.1). This must be done within the Code of Ethics for the Health Education Profression. When a conflict arises among individuals, groups, organizations, agencies or institutions, health education specialists must consider all issues and give priority to those that promote wellness and quality of living through principles of self-determination and freedom of choice for the individual. Health education specialists in the K-12 setting promote integrity in the delivery of health education. They respect the rights, dignity, confidentiality and worth of all people by adapting strategies and methods to meet the needs of diverse populations and communities. The health education specialist must demonstrate professionalism at all times staying up to date with best practices in the field and joining and supporting professional associations.

Health Care Setting: Health education specialists are expected to lead by example and demonstrate professional behavior and appropriate demeanor while on duty as they are representatives of the profession. It is the responsibility of all health education specialists to follow the 6 ethical principles outlined in the Code of Ethics for the Health Education Profession. It is expected that they also follow policies and regulations regarding workplace conduct and demeanor as warranted by their employers. Health education specialists working in health care settings may have access to highly confidential and personal health information. Therefore, they must be familiar with the Health Information Portability and Accountability Act (HIPAA) and abide by the principles of patient confidentiality. Health education specialists are expected to have cultural sensitivity and competency awareness skills, and advocate for diversity and inclusion. They must evaluate their own unconscious biases and demonstrate no bias to colleagues, clients, and the community they serve. Health education specialist professionals are accountable for their actions, decisions, and the impact of their practice. It is incumbent on all health education specialists to seek professional development opportunities for themselves so as to remain current in the field and provide professional development opportunities for any others they may supervise.

College/University Setting: Ethical behavior in all health education settings is guided by the Code of Ethics for the Health Education Proffression. The Code of Ethics applies to the college/university health education specialist when teaching, advising students, conducting and disseminating research (via presentations and publications) and service. Traits related to responsible practice include honesty, equity and fairness, cultural humility, preparation for practice and ongoing reflection. Professionalism involves behaving in a manner consistent with best practices and ethical behavior, staying up to date in the field, and taking the responsibility to further the health education profession. One's personal reputation and the reputation of the health education professions is dependent on ethical and professional behavior.

Worksite/Business Setting: Health education specialists' behavior is guided by the Code of Ethics for the Health Education Profession. In addition, there may be additional ethical guidelines related to the business function(s) of the worksite, the health education specialists' role in the organization, and/or statutory guidelines. For example, a health education specialist may have fiduciary responsibilities if they are part of the decision-making process related to the employer's health plan and medical benefits. There may also be vendor contractual obligations that govern aspects of a health education specialist's behavior. Every worksite has a unique culture and a set of either formal and/or informal standards of professional behavior that guide health education specialists. It is expected that the health education specialist will demonstrate professional behavior at all times within the cultural norms of the setting. The health education specialist will remain current and updated on the latest trends and initiatives in the field.

College/University Health Promotion Services Setting: Health education specialists in this setting adhere to the Code of Ethics for the Health Education Proffression as outlined by a variety of health and higher education professional organizations. Within this setting, health education specialists must practice cultural humility, inclusion, respect, and promote equity when working with diverse and changing priority populations of colleagues, employees, and students. They must adhere to ethical protocols and procedures, ensure privacy of data and files, and comply with federal laws and regulations. To do so they must engage in a variety of professional development opportunities and should participate in one or more professional associations.

Table 3.9
Health Education Specialist Practice Analysis II 2020 Model: Area of Responsibility VIII: Ethics and Professionalism

Area of Responsibility VIII: Ethics and Professionalism					
Entry-level Sub-competencies		**Advanced 1-level Sub-competencies**		**Advanced 2-level Sub-competencies**	
Competency 8.1 Practice in accordance with established ethical principles					
8.1.1	Apply professional codes of ethics and ethical principles throughout assessment, planning, implementation, evaluation and research, communication, consulting, and advocacy processes				
		8.1.2	Demonstrate ethical leadership, management, and behavior		
8.1.3	Comply with legal standards and regulatory guidelines in assessment, planning, implementation, evaluation and research, advocacy, management, communication, and reporting processes				
8.1.4	Promote health equity				
8.1.5	Use evidence-informed theories, models, and strategies				
8.1.6	Apply principles of cultural humility, inclusion, and diversity in all aspects of practice (e.g., Culturally and Linguistically Appropriate Services (CLAS) standards and culturally responsive pedagogy)				
Competency 8.2 Serve as an authoritative resource on health education and promotion					
		8.2.1	Evaluate personal and organizational capacity to provide consultation		

Area of Responsibility VIII: Ethics and Professionalism					
Entry-level Sub-competencies		Advanced 1-level Sub-competencies		Advanced 2-level Sub-competencies	
Competency 8.2 Serve as an authoritative resource on health education and promotion (continued)					
		8.2.2	Provide expert consultation, assistance, and guidance to individuals, groups, and organizations		
				8.2.3	Conduct peer reviews (e.g., manuscripts, abstracts, proposals, and tenure folios)
Competency 8.3 Engage in professional development to maintain and/or enhance proficiency					
8.3.1	Participate in professional associations, coalitions, and networks (e.g., serving on committees, attending conferences, and providing leadership)				
8.3.2	Participate in continuing education opportunities to maintain or enhance continuing competence				
8.3.3	Develop a career advancement plan				
8.3.4	Build relationships with other professionals within and outside the profession				
				8.3.5	Serve as a mentor
Competency 8.4 Promote the health education profession to stakeholders, the public, and others					
8.4.1	Explain the major responsibilities, contributions, and value of the health education specialist				
8.4.2	Explain the role of professional organizations and the benefits of participating in them				
8.4.3	Advocate for professional development for health education specialists				

SECTION III

SECTION III

Area of Responsibility VIII: Ethics and Professionalism				
Entry-level Sub-competencies		Advanced 1-level Sub-competencies		Advanced 2-level Sub-competencies
Competency 8.4 Promote the health education profession to stakeholders, the public, and others (continued)				
8.4.4	Educate others about the history of the profession, its current status, and its implications for professional practice			
8.4.5	Explain the role and benefits of credentialing (e.g., individual and program)			
		8.4.6	Develop presentations and publications that contribute to the profession	
		8.4.7	Engage in service to advance the profession	

The HESPA II 2020 is the fifth analysis of its kind to assure that qualified health education specialists have the knowledge and skills to educate and improve the health of the public. The first role delineation study was conducted from 1978 to 1981 and formed the basis for professional preparation, professional development, and the CHES® examination (Cleary, 1995). Next, from the CUP Model (NCHEC, SOPHE, & AAHE, 2006), common standards of practice were introduced in a hierarchical framework of entry-, advanced 1- and advanced 2- level Sub-competencies for health educators. The HEJA 2010 (NCHEC, SOPHE, & AAHE, 2010) added additional Sub-competencies and refined the hierarchical model. The HESPA I (NCHEC & SOPHE) 2015 added additional Competencies and Sub-competencies, introduced a terminology change from "health educator" to "health education specialist" and changed the title from "job analysis" to "practice analysis" to better reflect the breadth of the profession.

A variety of stakeholders used these models to more clearly define, develop, and apply the Competencies and Sub-competencies of the profession. Like the HESPA I 2015 Model, the HESPA II 2020 Model serves the profession in a number of ways. This time, the HESPA II 2020 Model includes the newly-validated Eight Areas of Responsibility and 35 Competencies, as well as 114 entry-level, 59 advanced 1-level, and 20 advanced 2-level Sub-competencies. The addition of the eighth Area of Responsibility, Ethics and Professionalism, emphasizes the overarching nature and importance of ethics in health education/promotion practice. The HESPA II 2020 Model also includes 145 verified Knowledge items used by health education specialists. The following text is presented to describe the potential applications and benefits of the HESPA II 2020 Model for selected stakeholder groups, including a set of formal recommendations to the profession endorsed by the boards of SOPHE, NCHEC, and CNHEO.

Health Education/Promotion Students

Often students find choosing a career path in health education to be a confusing process. This confusion may be particularly true for individuals entering a university system for the first time with limited exposure to the work settings associated with the wide variety of health education career options. Like its predecessors, the HESPA II 2020 Model offers useful information to students interested in a career in health education/promotion, including a basic understanding of the Competencies and Sub-competencies commonly used by health education specialists. The HESPA II 2020 Model also serves as a guide for students exploring the various work settings in which this understanding might be applied. Students considering a graduate degree in health education are better prepared to make the decision and choose a program if they are familiar with the entry- and advanced-level distinctions in the Model. The Model also allows students to compare the stated Competencies in other professions and understand professional distinctions in general.

Students enrolled in health education degree programs may use the Model as a guide for self-directed learning and assessment. Moreover, the Model may help students set personal achievement goals specific to each Area of Responsibility and, subsequently, to assess progress toward mastery of each Area. Students may use the Competencies and Sub-competencies as a guide for selecting and evaluating degree programs and specific courses, as well as for actively seeking opportunities to serve as volunteers, interns, and/or employees to gain experience in specific Areas of Responsibility. The

Section IV: Using the HESPA II 2020 Model

Model may be used as a framework in preparing for the national examination to become a CHES® or MCHES®. The framework also helps to create professional portfolios and résumés that reflect experiences and demonstrated abilities relevant to the profession.

College and University Health Education/Promotion Faculty

Faculty members of health education professional preparation programs may use the HESPA II 2020 Model for curriculum development, student mentorship, and program accreditation efforts. A Competency-based approach to curriculum development can enhance the marketability of program graduates and is an established standard for achieving formal approval/accreditation for health education programs. Faculty members and their students may benefit when expectations for student performance, faculty members' teaching, and mentorship are clearly defined within the Model framework. The Model is useful in developing program goals and objectives, course descriptions, syllabi and evaluation instruments, student handbooks, and specific guides for practica/internships, as well as portfolios and assessment tools for program approval and accreditation. The Model also may help faculty members to compare the stated competencies of other professional degrees offered by a university and develop program descriptions and marketing materials. Furthermore, the Model can serve as a guide for faculty members to communicate program needs to university administrators and to leverage resources and opportunities for program development or improvement. Faculty members are encouraged to seek and maintain CEPH or CAEP accreditation relevant to their degree programs and to conduct periodic reviews to assess and maintain relevance and currency in their programs (see Appendix D for matrices for analyzing curricula).

Health Education Practitioners and Researchers

Practicing health education specialists may use the HESPA II 2020 Model as a guide for professional development. Continuing education is not only a requirement for CHES® and MCHES® certifications but also essential for a practicing health education specialist to remain current, effective, and marketable in the field. The HESPA II 2020 Model is useful in helping practitioners monitor changes in Competencies and Sub-competencies as they emerge, self-assess areas of needed renewal and new skill development, select professional development opportunities directed toward current practices in the profession, and advocate to their employers for support of continuing education opportunities.

Researchers can use the HESPA II 2020 Model as a basis for conducting investigations that can improve the teaching of health education specialists or implementation science. Practitioners who are interested in obtaining an advanced degree, changing work settings and/or being promoted to more advanced-levels of practice will be better equipped to do so if they are aware of and skilled in the generic entry-level and relevant advanced-level Competencies represented in the Model. Practitioners can also use the HESPA II 2020 Model in writing resolutions, providing testimony, or authoring publications to advance the public's health or health education teaching, research and practice.

Professional Development Providers

Health education specialists are often required to demonstrate that they have completed some professional development as part of their employment responsibilities. Leaders of organizations and agencies that provide continuing education and professional development opportunities will benefit from using the HESPA II 2020 Model as a guide. For example, health education specialists often look to these organizations and agencies as a source for staying current in an evolving professional field. As the number of CHES® and MCHES® continue to grow, the demand for Competency-based professional development opportunities will increase. Opportunities to renew and develop new skills represented in the HESPA II 2020 Model will be critical to the future of a growing and evolving health education profession.

Other Professionals

The previously completed Role Delineation Project, CUP, HEJA 2010 and HESPA I 2015 Models have contributed to a growing understanding and appreciation for health education specialists among members of other health and non-health professions. Likewise, the HESPA II 2020 Model can be used to improve understanding of health education specialists and their valuable roles in health-related partnerships. The Model can be used to show others what health education specialists can contribute to policy, systems and environmental changes that help people improve and maintain their health.

Health Education/Promotion Employers

Most Competencies used by health education specialists are adaptable to a variety of work-related projects. Some Competencies enable a health education specialist to connect other health education specialists and communities together, as well as to achieve objectives in health-promoting partnerships. The HESPA II 2020 Model contains an updated, empirically verified description of current practice at three levels and supports employment of health education specialists. Employers are encouraged to use the HESPA II 2020 Model when developing position announcements and job descriptions, supporting and requiring professional development for their employed health education specialists, and evaluating employee performance. HESPA II 2020 Competencies and Sub-competencies in leadership and management can help employers maximize their operations. CHES® and MCHES® credentials reflect mastery of current entry- and advanced-level Areas of Responsibility, Competencies, and Sub-competencies and requires continued professional development to maintain the credentials.

Employers should hire individuals with these certifications.

Leaders of Professional Credentialing and Program Accreditation

The HESPA II 2020 Model serves as the standard for individual credentialing and program approval or accreditation. The HESPA II 2020 Model contains Eight Responsibilities instead of Seven and has some different Sub-competencies and Competencies than the CUP, HEJA 2010 or the HESPA I 2015 Models; therefore, it requires the development of specific items for the current CHES® and MCHES® examinations, as well as adjustments to criteria for program approval and accreditation. These changes enhance the profession's ability to assess and promote individual Competencies and program quality based on a more precise and expanded definition of Competencies and Sub-competencies. Inclusion of the entry-level Competencies at all levels of credentialing and accreditation and the addition of the advanced-level Competencies in criteria used for advanced-level credentialing and professional preparation will be important.

Policy Makers and Funding Organizations

Policy makers or organizational leaders may use the HESPA II 2020 Model in governmental and non-governmental settings to help establish organizational priorities or policies related to health education and social determinants of health. These decisions often impact the development of health programs and interventions, as well as the criteria for funding projects and research. The Competencies and Sub-competencies further clarify the distinctive role of health education specialists at entry- and advanced-levels of practice. The United States Department of Labor and the states implementing the Standard Occupational Classification system should use the HESPA II 2020 Model to collect data and monitor the job outlook for health education specialists.

SECTION IV

Implications for the Profession

The HESPA II 2020 Model has significant implications for professional preparation, certification, continuing education, and practice in the health education profession. In 2019, the TAG proposed twelve recommendations which were approved by the boards of SOPHE and NCHEC for using the HESPA II 2020 Model, which were later endorsed by the CNHEO. The recommendations build on earlier studies and reports for the field and reaffirm the following key principles: (a) health education is a single profession with common **roles** and responsibilities; (b) professional preparation in health education provides a health education specialist with knowledge and skills that form a foundation of generic Competencies; (c) accreditation is the primary quality assurance mechanism in higher education; and (d) the health education profession is responsible for assuring quality in professional preparation and practice.

Recommendations for Advancing the Profession

To continue to advance the profession, the following recommendations (NCHEC & SOPHE, 2019) provide a basis and direction for all future efforts:

1. Baccalaureate degree programs with a health education and promotion emphasis should prepare graduates to perform all entry-level Competencies and Sub-competencies within the Eight Areas of Responsibility. Additionally, curricula should incorporate the verified Knowledge items.

2. Master's programs with a health education and promotion emphasis should prepare graduates to perform all entry-level and advanced 1-level Competencies and Sub-competencies within the Eight Areas of Responsibility. Additionally, curricula should incorporate the verified Knowledge items.

3. Doctoral programs with a health education and promotion emphasis should prepare graduates to perform all entry-level, advanced 1-level and advanced 2-level Competencies and Sub-competencies within the Eight Areas of Responsibility. Additionally, curricula should incorporate the verified Knowledge items.

4. NCHEC should use all entry-level Competencies and Sub-competencies within the Eight Areas of Responsibility as the basis for the Certified Health Education Specialist (CHES®) examination. Additionally, verified Knowledge items will be utilized in the development of exam questions.

5. NCHEC should use all entry-level, advanced 1-level and advanced 2-level Competencies and Sub-competencies within the Eight Areas of Responsibility as the basis for the advanced-level Master Certified Health Education Specialist (MCHES®) examination. Additionally, verified Knowledge items should be utilized in the development of exam questions.

6. Entry-level and advanced-level Competencies and Sub-competencies within the Eight Areas of Responsibility and the verified Knowledge items should serve as the basis for professional development and continuing education for the health education and promotion profession.

7.   Accrediting agencies and approval bodies should recognize the Eight Areas of Responsibility, Competencies, and Sub-competencies as the basis for quality assurance of health education professional preparation programs in all workforce settings.

8.   The HESPA II 2020 hierarchical model should be used as the basis for communicating about the Responsibilities and Competencies of all health education specialists to public and private employers, national/state/local government agencies, health insurers, health professionals, and other stakeholders.

9.   Public and private employers should hire certified health education specialists and utilize the HESPA II 2020 Responsibilities and Competencies in developing job descriptions and evaluating the performance of their health education and promotion workforce.

10. Public and private employers should provide support for professional development and continuing education offerings aligned with the latest HESPA II 2020 Responsibilities and Competencies, as a means of promoting continuing competency of their health education and promotion workforce.

11. Health education specialists at all levels of education and experience should abide by ethical principles and practices in alignment with the HESPA II 2020 hierarchical model.

12. As the profession moves forward, all those practicing health education and promotion should obtain and maintain certification as a health education specialist.

Profession-wide support of these 12 recommendations can significantly impact the future of the health education profession. For example, NCHEC leaders are using the HESPA II 2020 Model and verified Knowledge items to update the CHES® and MCHES® examinations effective in 2022 and moving forward. SOPHE used the HESPA II 2020 Model as the basis for developing standards for school health educator teacher preparation, recognized under CAEP. Professional development and continuing education opportunities may be planned for the three different levels of practice. As with previous practice analyses, the HESPA II 2020 Model serves as a guide for future Competency updates. The regular, periodic revalidation of the health education Areas of Responsibility, Competencies, and Sub-competencies is a necessary process to ensure that certification, preparation, and professional development are based on the needs of current workforce practice. Ideally this revalidation process will be completed every five years.

Notes

Section V

Changes in the Areas of Responsibility: Competencies and Sub-competencies of Health Education Specialists from 1985 to 2020

HESPA II 2020 marks the 35th year since the publication of *A Framework for the Development of Competency-based Curricula for Entry-level Health Educators* (Cleary, 1995), a document which outlined the Seven Areas of Responsibility and signified the first established role of entry-level health education specialists and their related scope of practice. The HESPA II 2020 Model presents the fourth series of changes made to that original framework and represents the emerging changes in current practice. Table 5.1 illustrates the progression of the Areas of Responsibility. In 1985, the profession began with Seven Areas of Responsibility (Cleary, 1995). Three graduate-level areas (i.e., Areas VIII-X) were added in 1999 (NCHEC, AAHE, & SOPHE, 1999). In 2006, the original Seven Areas of Responsibility from 1985 and three graduate-level Areas from 1999 were combined into an updated Seven Areas of Responsibility (Gilmore, et al., 2005). The profession further refined the Seven Areas of Responsibility in 2010 and revalidated the Seven Areas of Responsibility in the HESPA I 2015 Model (Doyle, et al., 2012; NCHEC & SOPHE, 2015). In HESPA II 2020, the Areas of Responsibility were expanded and validated into eight areas, as shown in Table 5.1. Although the framework has evolved over the past three and a half decades, the Areas of Responsibility remain largely intact. The current model represents both the stability and the advancement of the profession.

The three-tiered hierarchical framework of entry- and advanced-level practice that emerged in the CUP Model has now been revalidated three times through the HEJA 2010, HESPA I 2015, and HESPA II 2020 Models. A large number of Competencies and Sub-competencies have also been revalidated. However, as was found in the previous validation studies, the HESPA II 2020 Model reveals the need for wording changes, the reassignment of some Competencies and Sub-competencies, and the addition of new Competencies and Sub-competencies to more accurately reflect the evolving practice of entry- and advanced-level health education specialists. The descriptions below include a brief overview of changes made in the HESPA II 2020 Model compared to the HESPA I 2015 Model. A more detailed analysis of these changes appears in the grid provided in Appendix B.1.

EIGHT AREAS OF RESPONSIBILITY

The outcomes of the HESPA II 2020 resulted in four primary changes for the Areas of Responsibility: the conversion to Eight Areas of Responsibility; the renaming of some Areas of Responsibility; the removal of health education/promotion from all Areas of Responsibility to make them more succinct; and a reordering of the Areas of Responsibility. The foundation of the Eight Areas of Responsibility validated in the current study is the Seven Areas of Responsibility established and verified in the CUP, HEJA 2010, and HESPA I 2015 Models. The addition of an eighth Area of Responsibility indicates an evolution and reprioritization of the Competencies and Sub-competencies within the HESPA I 2015 *Area of Responsibility VII: Communicate, Promote, and Advocate for Health, Health Education, and the Profession*. This Area of Responsibility was split into two: 1) *Communication*, prompted by the rapid expansion of communication strategies and technology, and 2) *Advocacy*, acknowledging the increased emphasis of advocacy to effectively address the socio-ecologic factors impacting the health of individuals, communities, and populations.

HESPA II 2020 also validated another new Area of Responsibility: *Ethics and Professionalism*. Competencies and Sub-competencies relating to ethics were found in all Seven Areas of Responsibility in the HESPA I 2015 Model. The Health Education Practice Panel (HEPP) felt it important to consolidate these Competencies and Sub-competencies into one Area of Responsibility emphasizing the overarching nature and importance of ethics in health education/promotion practice. Since there are only Eight Areas of Responsibility in the current model, it is evident that the addition of this Area of Responsibility included the removal of another. The HESPA II 2020 Model reclassified the Competencies and Sub-competencies found within the HESPA I 2015 *Area of Responsibility VI: Serve as a Health Education/Promotion Resource Person*. The Competencies and Sub-competencies in this Area of Responsibility are housed in multiple Areas of Responsibility in the HESPA II 2020 Model, primarily *Area VIII: Ethics and Professionalism, Area VII: Leadership and Management*, and *Area VI: Communication*.

Name modifications to the Areas of Responsibility were made to more accurately reflect current and emerging health education practice. For example, the HESPA I 2015 Model Area of Responsibility *Administer and Manage Health Education/Promotion* was expanded to *Leadership and Management* in the current model. The previous model Area of Responsibility *Assess Needs, Resources, and Capacity for Health Education/Promotion* was altered to *Assessment of Needs and Capacity*. The term "capacity" encompasses resources, thus the word resources was removed due to its redundancy. The most notable nomenclature changes in the updated model are in the truncation of the Areas of Responsibility. The HESPA I 2015 Model replaced the term health education with health education/promotion in the names of the Areas of Responsibility to reflect that health education practice had extended beyond the individual level. In the past five years, health promotion as a foundational practice of health education specialists has become fully integrated, as evidenced by the emphasis of socio-ecologic concepts validated in the HESPA II 2020 Competencies and Sub-competencies. Thus, health education/

promotion is implied within the Areas of Responsibility for health education specialists. Although health education/promotion terminology has been removed from the names of the Areas of Responsibility, the health education/promotion terminology remains in the Competencies and Sub-competencies.

The last change in the HESPA II 2020 Model relating to the Areas of Responsibility is in the ordering. The first five Areas of Responsibility encompass specific, distinct aspects of health education/promotion practice. These are *Assessment of Needs and Capacity*; *Planning*; *Implementation*; *Evaluation and Research*; and *Advocacy*. The remaining three are overarching and are integrated into the first five. These are *Communication*; *Leadership and Management*; and *Ethics and Professionalism*.

COMPETENCIES AND SUB-COMPETENCIES

The Competencies and Sub-competencies were also updated during this practice analysis. The HESPA II 2020 HEPP worked diligently to streamline the Competencies and Sub-competencies to decrease redundancy and increase utility for those developing professional preparation curricula, providing continuing education, and writing the certification examinations. The HEPP also helped clarify many of the Competencies and Sub-competencies through the addition of examples. For instance, examples are included in *Area V: Advocacy 5.2.8 Specify strategies, a timeline, and roles and responsibilities to address the proposed policy, system, or environmental change (e.g., develop ongoing relationships with decision makers and stakeholders, use social media, register others to vote, and seek political appointment)*. Another example where the Sub-competency is clarified is in *Area VI: Communication 6.1.2 Identify the assets, needs, and characteristics of the audience(s) that affect communication and message design (e.g., literacy levels, language, culture, and cognitive and perceptual abilities)*.

Section V: Changes in the Areas of Responsibility: Competencies and Sub-competencies of Health Education Specialists from 1985 to 2020

Table 5.1
Comparison of Areas of Responsibility (1985 – 2020)

Entry-Level Framework (1985)	Graduate-Level Framework (1999)	CUP Model (2006)	HEJA Model (2010)	HESPA I Model (2015)	HESPA II Model (2020)
I. Assessing individual and community needs for health education	I. Assessing individual and community needs for health education	I. Assess individual and community needs for health education	I. Assess needs, assets, and capacity for health education	I. Assess needs, resources, and capacity for health education/promotion	I. Assessment of needs and capacity
II. Planning effective health education programs	II. Planning effective health education programs	II. Plan health education strategies, interventions, and programs	II. Plan health education	II. Plan health education/ promotion	II. Planning
III. Implementing health education programs	III. Implementing health education programs	III. Implement health education strategies, interventions, and programs	III. Implement health education	III. Implement health education/promotion	III. Implementation
IV. Evaluating the effectiveness of health education programs	IV. Evaluating effectiveness of health education programs	IV. Conduct evaluation and research related to health education	IV. Conduct evaluation and research related to health education	IV. Conduct evaluation and research related to health education/promotion	IV. Evaluation and research
V. Coordinating provision of health education services	V. Coordinating provision of health education services	V. Administer health education strategies, interventions, and programs	V. Administer and manage health education	V. Administer and manage health education/promotion	V. Advocacy
VI. Acting as a resource person in health education	VI. Acting as a resource person in health education	VI. Serve as a health education resource person	VI. Serve as a health education resource person	VI. Serve as a health education/promotion resource person	VI. Communication
VII. Communicating health and health education needs, concerns and resources	VII. Communicating health and health education needs, concerns and resources	VII. Communicate and advocate for health and health education	VII. Communicate and advocate for health and health education	VII. Communicate, promote, and advocate for health, health education/ promotion and the profession	VII. Leadership and Management
	VIII. Applying appropriate research principles and techniques in health education				VIII. Ethics and Professionalism
	IX. Administering health education programs				
	X. Advancing the profession of health education				

Note. Adapted from *Overview of the National Health Educator Competencies Update Project, 1998-2004* (Gilmore et. al., 2005), *A Competency-Based Framework for Health Education Specialists – 2010* (National Commission for Health Education Credentialing Inc., Society for Public Health Education, & American Association for Health Education, 2010), and *A Competency-Based Framework for Health Education Specialists – 2015* (National Commission for Health Education Credentialing, Inc. & Society for Public Health Education, 2015).

Section V: Changes in the Areas of Responsibility: Competencies and Sub-competencies of Health Education Specialists from 1985 to 2020

The number of Competencies and Sub-competencies are displayed in Table 5.2a (HESPA I 2015 Model) and Table 5.2b (HESPA II 2020 Model). Notice the decrease in the total number of Sub-competencies from 258 in the HESPA I 2015 Model to 193 in the HESPA II 2020 Model. The Sub-competencies also differ according to their levels of practice within the HESPA I 2015 and HESPA II 2020 Models. Of the 258 Sub-competencies in the HESPA I 2015 Model, 141 (54.7%) were validated at the entry-level, 76 (29.5%) at the advanced 1-level, and 41(15.9%) at the advanced 2-level. Of the 193 Sub-competencies in the HESPA II 2020 Model, 114 (59.17%) were validated at the entry-level, 59 (30.6%) were validated at the advanced 1-level, and 20 (10.4 %) were validated at the advanced 2-level. Although the number of Competencies and Sub-competencies has decreased, all of the topical areas covered in the HESPA I 2015 Competencies and Sub-competencies are represented within the HESPA II 2020 Model. It is important to note that only Sub-competencies, and not Competencies, are classified as entry-level (or generic), advanced 1-level, or advanced 2-level.

Table 5.2a
Competencies and Sub-competencies at Each Level of Practice for the HESPA I 2015 Model

Areas of Responsibility	Competencies	Total Sub-competencies	Entry-level Sub-competencies	Advanced 1-level Sub-competencies	Advanced 2-level Sub-competencies
Area I – Assess Needs, Resources, and Capacity for Health Education/Promotion	7	33	30	3	0
Area II – Plan Health Education/Promotion	5	34	28	6	0
Area III – Implement Health Education/Promotion	4	29	21	8	0
Area IV – Conduct Evaluation and Research related to Health Education/Promotion	7	57	9	10	38
Area V – Administer and Manage Health Education/Promotion	6	51	18	33	0
Area VI – Serve as a Health Education/Promotion Resource Person	3	16	5	11	0
Area VII – Communicate, Promote, and Advocate for Health, Health Education/Promotion and the Profession	4	38	30	5	3
Total	**36**	**258**	**141**	**76**	**41**

Section V: Changes in the Areas of Responsibility: Competencies and Sub-competencies of Health Education Specialists from 1985 to 2020

There were six Competencies within the HESPA II 2020 model in which all Sub-competencies validated at the advanced level. These were: *4.2 Design research studies; 4.5 Use findings; 7.3 Manage human resources; 7.4 Manage fiduciary and material resources; 7.5 Conduct strategic planning with appropriate stakeholders; and 8.2 Serve as an authoritative resource in health education and promotion.* Advanced-level Sub-competencies of the HESPA II 2020 Model can be found within all Areas of Responsibility but are concentrated in *Area of Responsibility IV: Evaluation and Research* and *Area of Responsibility VII: Leadership and Management.* The Sub-competencies validated at the advanced 2-level of practice primarily relate to planning research, collecting and analyzing data, working with data collection instruments, interpreting and disseminating research findings, and mentoring less experienced health education specialists. The Sub-competencies

validated at advanced 1-level predominantly relate to evaluation and management.

The three distinct levels of practice initially established through the CUP study were reverified in the HEJA 2010, HESPA I 2015, and HESPA II 2020 Models. These are entry-level, advanced 1-level, and advanced 2-level. Consistent with earlier practice analyses, these practice levels are hierarchical in the HESPA II 2020 Model. The Sub-competencies in the advanced 1-level include generic Sub-competencies at the entry-level and Sub-competencies specific to the advanced 1-level practice. The Sub-competencies in the advanced 2-level include generic (entry-level) Sub-competencies, advanced 1-level Sub-competencies, and an additional set of Sub-competencies specific to advanced 2-level practice.

Table 5.2b
Competencies and Sub-competencies at Each Level of Practice for the HESPA II 2020 Model

Areas of Responsibility	Competencies	Total Sub-competencies	Entry-level Sub-competencies	Advanced 1-level Sub-competencies	Advanced 2-level Sub-competencies
Area I – Assessment of Needs and Capacity	4	25	22	3	0
Area II – Planning	4	19	11	8	0
Area III - Implementation	3	16	15	1	0
Area IV – Evaluation and Research	5	37	6	16	15
Area V – Advocacy	4	18	16	2	0
Area VI – Communication	6	26	24	1	1
Area VII – Leadership and Management	5	31	6	23	2
Area VIII – Ethics and Professionalism	4	21	14	5	2
Total	**35**	**193**	**114**	**59**	**20**

Section V: Changes in the Areas of Responsibility: Competencies and Sub-competencies of Health Education Specialists from 1985 to 2020

AREA OF RESPONSIBILITY I:
Assessment of Needs and Capacity

In Area of Responsibility I: *Assessment of Needs and Capacity*, there is a close alignment with the Competencies and Sub-competencies found in HESPA I 2015. The change in the number of Competencies from the HESPA I 2015 Model to the HESPA II 2020 Model decreased from seven to four respectively. The fewer number resulted from the consolidation of Competencies. For example, HESPA I 2015 *Competencies 1.2 Access existing information and data related to health* and *1.3 Collect primary data to determine needs* have been combined to the HESPA II 2020 *1.2 Obtain primary data, secondary data, and other evidence-informed sources*.

The total number of Sub-competencies in Area of Responsibility I decreased from 33 in the HESPA I 2015 Model to 25 in the HESPA II 2020 Model. Once again, this change resulted from the combination of multiple Sub-competencies from HESPA I 2015 Model in the HESPA II 2020 Model. For example, five HESPA I 2015 Sub-competencies in Competencies 1.4 and 1.5 relating to factors that impact health and learning such as knowledge, attitudes, beliefs, behaviors, and skills (i.e., Sub-competencies 1.4.1, 1.4.2, 1.5.2, 1.5.3, and 1.5.4) were consolidated to form the HESPA II 2020 Sub-competency *1.3.2 Determine the knowledge, attitudes, beliefs, skills and behaviors that impact the health and health literacy of the priority population(s)*. One new Sub-competency found in *Area I Assessment of Needs and Capacity* is *1.4.3 Summarize the capacity of priority population(s) to meet the needs of the priority population(s)*. See Appendix B.1 for a detailed comparison of the HESPA I 2015 and HESPA II 2020 Competencies and Sub-competencies.

AREA OF RESPONSIBILITY II:
Planning

There is also a close alignment of the Competencies and Sub-competencies in Area of Responsibility II: *Planning*, with the HESPA I 2015 *Plan Health Education/ Promotion*. The number of Competencies in this Area of Responsibility changed from five to four, while the number of Sub-competencies decreased from 34 in the HESPA I 2015 Model to 19 in the HESPA II 2020 Model due to the streamlining of Competencies and Sub-competencies. HESPA I 2015 *Competencies 2.4 Develop a plan for the delivery of health education/ promotion* and *2.5 Address factors that influence implementation of health education/promotion* were combined to form HESPA II 2020 *Competency 2.4 Develop plans and materials for implementation and evaluation*. One new Sub-competency was added to the Area of Responsibility. It is *2.4.4 Plan for evaluation and dissemination of results*, conveying the relationship between planning and evaluation processes.

AREA OF RESPONSIBILITY III:
Implementation

Area of Responsibility III: *Implementation* had very few changes from the previous model. Two of the HESPA I 2015 Competencies were combined, resulting in a change from four Competencies in HESPA I 2015 to three in HESPA II 2020. The number of Sub-competencies decreased from 29 in HESPA I 2015 to 16 in HESPA II 2020. A notable change is the inclusion of the term fidelity to two Sub-competencies, drawing attention to the importance of fidelity in increasing the likelihood of positive outcomes.

AREA OF RESPONSIBILITY IV:
Evaluation and Research

Area of Responsibility IV: *Evaluation and Research decreased* from seven Competencies and 57 Sub-competencies in the HESPA I 2015 Model to five Competencies and 37 Sub-competencies in the

Section V: Changes in the Areas of Responsibility: Competencies and Sub-competencies of Health Education Specialists from 1985 to 2020

HESPA II 2020 Model through consolidation as seen in the other Areas of Responsibility. Sub-competencies within this Area of Responsibility remained in this Area from the HESPA I 2015 and HESPA II 2020 Models. Two new Sub-competencies were added: *4.2.3 Use a logic model and/or theory for research* and *4.4.5 Identify implications for practice*. Both of these Sub-competencies relate to research and were exclusive to evaluation in the HESPA I 2015 Model. Forty-eight of the 57 Sub-competencies of Evaluation and Research fall within the purview of advanced-level practice in HESPA I 2015. In addition, 15 of the 16 advanced-level Sub-competencies in HESPA I 2015 correspond with advanced 2-level practice in HESPA II 2020.

AREA OF RESPONSIBILITY V:
Advocacy

Advocacy was validated as a standalone Area of Responsibility in HESPA II 2020 and represents an increased emphasis on advocacy in the health education profession. Utilization of coalitions as a method of change is more overtly included in this Area within HESPA II 2020. Included also is sustaining the relationships for systems change. There are four Competencies and 18 Sub-competencies. Two of the four Competencies found within this Area of Responsibility were new: *5.2 Engage coalitions and stakeholders in addressing the health issue and planning advocacy efforts* and *5.4 Evaluate Advocacy*. Sub-competencies new to the HESPA II 2020 Model are *5.2.1 Identify existing coalitions and stakeholders in addressing the health issue and planning advocacy efforts* and *5.4.2 Use the evaluation results to inform next steps*.

AREA OF RESPONSIBILITY VI:
Communication

Communication was also validated as a standalone Area of Responsibility in HESPA II 2020. This Area of Responsibility has six Competencies and 26 Sub-competencies, whereas the HESPA I 2015 Model had only one Competency and eight Sub-competencies dedi-

cated solely to Communication. Many of the Competencies and Sub-competencies in the current model were reclassified from other Areas of Responsibility (primarily from *Areas VI: Serve as a Health Education/ Promotion Resource Person* and *VII: Communicate, Promote, and Advocate for Health, Health Education/ Promotion, and the Profession* in the HESPA I 2015 Model.) The new Competencies and Sub-competencies relate communication as a unique process that requires segmentation, employing media literacy processes, and materials specifically designed for communication. Communication is also considered to be embedded in all aspects of health education/ promotion practice. Effective communication using interpersonal as well as technology skills also has increased emphasis in HESPA II 2020. The Sub-competencies are considered fundamental to all levels of health education and promotion practice as 24 of the 26) Sub-competencies validated as generic (i.e., at the entry-level).

AREA OF RESPONSIBILITY VII:
Leadership and Management

Area of Responsibility VII: *Leadership and Management* in the HESPA II 2020 Model incorporates many reclassified Competencies and Sub-competencies from the HESPA I 2015 *Areas of Responsibility V: Administer and Manage Health Education/Promotion* and *Area VI: Serve as a Health Education/Promotion Resource Person*. It has five Competencies and 31 Sub-competencies. Of the 31 Sub-competencies, 25 validated at advanced-level practice. These Sub-competencies focus on managing relationships; training others to engage in health education/ promotion activities; managing human, fiduciary, and material resources; and facilitating strategic planning.

Section V: Changes in the Areas of Responsibility: Competencies and Sub-competencies of Health Education Specialists from 1985 to 2020

SECTION V

AREA OF RESPONSIBILITY VIII:
Ethics and Professionalism

The last Area of Responsibility Area VIII: *Ethics and Professionalism* is new as a responsibility, but most of the Competencies and Sub-competencies for this responsibility were integrated throughout the various Responsibilities in previous versions. Ethics and Professionalism is overarching and influences all aspects of health education/promotion practice. Its foundational essence is emphasized by its placement in the Areas of Responsibility. It is not an afterthought, but a required condition of being a health education specialist. Ethics and Professionalism has four Competencies and 21 Sub-competencies. Two of the four Competencies were reclassified with revision from other HESPA I 2015 Areas of Responsibility. One was the reclassification of HESPA I 2015 Competency *7.4 Promote the health education profession* to HESPA II 2020 *8.4 Promote the health education profession to stakeholders, the public, and others*. The variation in wording emphasizes the importance of educating those with whom the profession interacts. The other was a reclassification and rewording of *6.3 Provide advice and consultation on health education/promotion* to HESPA II 2020 *8.2 Serve as an authoritative resource on health education and promotion*. The newly worded Competency includes Sub-competencies that convey assessment of capacity and higher-level service to the profession (e.g., peer review). All of the Sub-competencies for 8.2 validated as advanced-level practice.

One of the new Competencies resulted from an elevation of a HESPA I 2015 Sub-competency *7.4.8 Develop and implement a professional development plan* to the HESPA II 2020 Competency *8.3 Engage in professional development to maintain and enhance proficiency*. The elevation relates to the continuous nature of the Competency. The other new Competency *8.1 Practice in accordance with established ethical principles* emphasizes the ethical obligations that health education specialists have with their employers, clients, peers, funders, and the overall profession.

The Sub-competencies in *Competency 8.1 relating to ethical practice* consolidate many re-classified HESPA I 2015 Sub-competencies. For example, *8.1.1 Apply professional codes of ethics and ethical principles throughout assessment, planning, implementation, evaluation, research, communication, consulting, and advocacy processes* represents a consolidation of 11 HESPA I 2015 Sub-competencies from six different HESPA I 2015 Areas of Responsibility. Two new Sub-competencies appear in this Area of Responsibility: *8.1.2 Demonstrate ethical leadership, management, and behavior* and *8.1.4 Promote health equity*.

Section VI

Core Knowledge Items

The ability to effectively perform a professional Competency is dependent in part on the mastery of relevant knowledge. However, clearly defining knowledge that is essential and generic to a Competency-based framework can be a challenge. The process of integrating a knowledge-based survey into a health education/promotion job analysis was first completed during HEJA 2010. This process was undertaken to identify and verify core Knowledge items for use in various aspects of professional preparation, credentialing, and professional development. A similar process was repeated with HESPA I 2015 and again with HESPA II 2020 because the verified core Knowledge items have been useful to those creating professional preparation programs, continuing education opportunities, and to those responsible for creating the certification examinations.

The previous Knowledge list was augmented with emerging areas of knowledge. The topics were organized into 10 conceptually related topic areas and included in the HESPA II 2020 survey. The same 4-point scale used to rate the Sub-competencies was adopted for rating the Knowledge items. Participants were asked to answer the following question: How frequently did you use the knowledge in your job as a health education specialist during the past 12 months? Respondents were asked to answer with one of the following: Not at all, Occasionally (less than once a month), Frequently (at least once each month), Very Frequently (at least once each week). Respondents were also asked to answer "How important is the Knowledge statement to your work as a health education specialist? The answer choices were "Not Important," "Minimally Important," "Moderately Important," and "Highly Important." After analysis, 145 of the 149 Knowledge statements were verified, and these statements have been included in the list provided on the following pages. Additional information about the validation process is in Section II of this publication.

After the Knowledge items were verified, a volunteer team of health education specialists with expertise in Competency development and credentialing reviewed each Knowledge item and assigned it to at least one of the Eight Areas of Responsibility in the HESPA II 2020 Model. Table 6.1 contains the Knowledge items (n=145) listed by conceptually related topics with the specific Area(s) to which each item was assigned designated by a ◆ in the table. This table can be used by university faculty who teach courses to which one or more of the Competencies and Sub-competencies under any of the Eight Areas of Responsibility have been assigned. The course instructor should ensure that the designated knowledge is addressed in the assigned course so students will be equipped with the knowledge needed to address related Competencies. Knowledge items are also used by continuing education providers whose programs support ongoing proficiency in the profession, and by associations to ensure the content provided in professional conferences are aligned to practice. Individual practitioners can also use the table as a guide for understanding and addressing needed knowledge bases when preparing for certification examinations or in self-guided professional development efforts. While the certification examinations are based on the Areas of Responsibility, Competencies, and Sub-competencies, and not on the Knowledge items, the people who write questions for the CHES® and MCHES® exams refer to the Knowledge items to help frame the context for questions that are then tied to the Competencies and Sub-competencies.

These 145 verified Knowledge items should not be considered an exhaustive representation of all essential core knowledge, and some items on the list may overlap in some ways, yet, each item on the list was empirically validated as essential to the work of health education specialists who participated in the study.

Additional research in future practice analyses is recommended to further explore and develop the broad knowledge base that is both generic and essential to the practice of health education specialists.

Table 6.1
Validated Knowledge Items by Topic and Area of Responsibility

	Knowledge of: **HEALTH EDUCATION PROFESSION**	Assessment of Needs and Capacity **Area I**	Planning **Area II**	Implementation **Area III**	Evaluation and Research **Area IV**	Advocacy **Area V**	Communication **Area VI**	Leadership and Management **Area VII**	Ethics and Professionalism **Area VIII**
1	Health education laws, rules, regulations (e.g., privacy, HIPAA, ACA, FERPA, ESSA, ADA, OSHA, GINA)	◆	◆	◆	◆	◆	◆	◆	◆
2	Health education history								◆
3	Health education and health promotion terminology	◆	◆	◆	◆	◆	◆	◆	◆
4	Health education framework (e.g., assessment, planning, implementation, evaluation)	◆	◆	◆	◆	◆	◆	◆	◆
5	Health education specialist role and responsibilities								◆
6	Health education professional preparation							◆	◆
7	Credentialing for individual practitioners, programs, and organizations in all settings (e.g., accreditation, licensure/certification)								◆
8	Health education professional associations								◆
9	Health education practice settings								◆
10	School health education standards	◆	◆	◆	◆				◆

Section VI: Core Knowledge Items

Knowledge of: **HEALTH EDUCATION PROFESSION**	Assessment of Needs and Capacity — Area I	Planning — Area II	Implementation — Area III	Evaluation and Research — Area IV	Advocacy — Area V	Communication — Area VI	Leadership and Management — Area VII	Ethics and Professionalism — Area VIII
11	School health education curriculum guidance (e.g., CDC Characteristics of an Effective Health Education Curricula)	◆	◆	◆	◆			◆	◆
12	Roles and responsibilities of inter-professional team members, including paraprofessionals							◆	◆
13	Professional development and continuing competence								◆
Knowledge of: **THEORIES AND TECHNIQUES**	Area I	Area II	Area III	Area IV	Area V	Area VI	Area VII	Area VIII
14	Education and learning theories		◆	◆			◆	◆	◆
15	Andragogy: principles and methods	◆	◆	◆			◆	◆	◆
16	Pedagogy: principles and methods	◆	◆	◆			◆	◆	◆
17	Health literacy, linguistics, and health numeracy	◆	◆	◆	◆		◆		◆
18	Curriculum development	◆	◆		◆			◆	◆
19	Training principles and methods	◆	◆	◆			◆	◆	◆
20	Lesson planning	◆	◆	◆	◆		◆		◆
21	Commonly used resources in health education (e.g., The Community Guide, Community Toolbox, School Health Index)	◆	◆	◆	◆	◆	◆	◆	◆
22	Cultural humility, inclusion, and diversity (e.g., sexual orientation, diverse learners, ethnicity, race)	◆	◆	◆	◆	◆	◆	◆	◆
23	Culturally and Linguistically Appropriate Services (CLAS) Standards	◆	◆	◆	◆	◆	◆	◆	◆

SECTION VI

Section VI: Core Knowledge Items

Knowledge of: THEORIES AND TECHNIQUES	Assessment of Needs and Capacity Area I	Planning Area II	Implementation Area III	Evaluation and Research Area IV	Advocacy Area V	Communication Area VI	Leadership and Management Area VII	Ethics and Professionalism Area VIII
24 Goals and SMART objectives		◆		◆		◆	◆	
25 Bloom's taxonomy		◆		◆		◆	◆	
26 Evidence-informed practice	◆	◆	◆	◆	◆	◆	◆	◆
27 Logic models	◆	◆	◆	◆	◆	◆	◆	◆
28 Behavior change theories, models, principles, and methods	◆	◆	◆	◆		◆		◆
29 Organization change theory		◆	◆				◆	
30 Health coaching principles and methods						◆		◆
31 Group facilitation principles and methods	◆	◆	◆	◆	◆	◆	◆	◆
32 Classroom management principles and methods			◆			◆		◆
33 Consulting and technical assistance							◆	◆
34 Mentoring principles and methods							◆	◆
35 Meeting planning and facilitation					◆		◆	
36 Strategic planning principles and methods (e.g., School/District Improvement Plan, results-based accountability, community health improvement plan)							◆	◆
37 Concepts related to mission and vision statements		◆			◆		◆	◆
38 Program implementation principles and practices (e.g., implementation science)			◆	◆			◆	◆

SECTION VI

Knowledge of: THEORIES AND TECHNIQUES	Assessment of Needs and Capacity Area I	Planning Area II	Implementation Area III	Evaluation and Research Area IV	Advocacy Area V	Communication Area VI	Leadership and Management Area VII	Ethics and Professionalism Area VIII
39 Strategies for participant recruitment, engagement, and retention	◆	◆	◆	◆	◆	◆	◆	◆
40 Program sustainability		◆	◆	◆			◆	◆
41 Program planning models, principles, and practices	◆	◆					◆	◆
42 Approaches to include Health in All Policies	◆	◆			◆		◆	◆
43 Determinants of health	◆	◆						◆
44 Health disparities	◆	◆	◆	◆	◆	◆	◆	◆
45 Social justice and health equity	◆	◆	◆	◆	◆	◆	◆	◆
46 Systems change theories (e.g., Socio-Ecological approach)	◆	◆	◆			◆	◆	◆
47 Whole School, Whole Community, Whole Child Model	◆	◆	◆	◆	◆	◆	◆	◆
48 Technology used in the delivery of health education (e.g., distance learning, and presentation software)		◆	◆	◆	◆	◆	◆	◆
49 Technology used in the management of health education and health education data	◆	◆	◆	◆	◆	◆	◆	◆
Knowledge of: ETHICS ACROSS ALL ASPECTS OF THE PROFESSION	Area I	Area II	Area III	Area IV	Area V	Area VI	Area VII	Area VIII
50 Ethical principles and responsibilities	◆	◆	◆	◆	◆	◆	◆	◆
51 Professional Code of Ethics	◆	◆	◆	◆	◆	◆	◆	◆
52 Ethical leadership and management principles and practices							◆	◆

SECTION VI

Section VI: Core Knowledge Items

Knowledge of: **ETHICS ACROSS ALL ASPECTS OF THE PROFESSION**	Assessment of Needs and Capacity Area I	Planning Area II	Implementation Area III	Evaluation and Research Area IV	Advocacy Area V	Communication Area VI	Leadership and Management Area VII	Ethics and Professionalism Area VIII
53 Ethical research and evaluation principles and practices				◆				◆
54 Ethical principles related to fundraising and advocacy					◆			◆
Knowledge of: **CAPACITY AND COMMUNITY BUILDING**	Area I	Area II	Area III	Area IV	Area V	Area VI	Area VII	Area VIII
55 Capacity building principles and methods	◆	◆	◆		◆		◆	◆
56 Coalitions principles and practices	◆	◆	◆		◆		◆	◆
57 Collaboration principles and methods	◆	◆	◆	◆	◆	◆	◆	◆
58 Community engagement principles and methods (e.g., school wellness councils, worksite wellness councils, patient-family advisory councils)	◆	◆			◆		◆	◆
59 Community organizing principles, methods, theories and models		◆	◆		◆		◆	◆
Knowledge of: **SYSTEMS**	Area I	Area II	Area III	Area IV	Area V	Area VI	Area VII	Area VIII
60 US health care system		◆			◆		◆	◆
61 Global health care systems		◆			◆		◆	◆
62 US public health system		◆			◆		◆	◆
63 Global public health systems		◆			◆		◆	◆
64 Health care payment models							◆	◆
65 US education system		◆			◆		◆	◆
66 Electronic health/medical records principles, laws, and ethics	◆			◆			◆	◆

SECTION VI

Section VI: Core Knowledge Items

Knowledge of: SYSTEMS	Assessment of Needs and Capacity — Area I	Planning — Area II	Implementation — Area III	Evaluation and Research — Area IV	Advocacy — Area V	Communication — Area VI	Leadership and Management — Area VII	Ethics and Professionalism — Area VIII
67 Information technology and database management	◆			◆			◆	◆
68 Data analytics and informatics	◆	◆		◆			◆	◆
69 Health information security principles			◆				◆	◆
70 Nonprofit boards, governance, laws, practice, and by-laws	◆	◆	◆	◆	◆	◆	◆	◆
71 Role of philanthropy and foundations in improving health	◆	◆					◆	◆

Knowledge of: RESEARCH, EVALUATION, AND DATA COLLECTION	Area I	Area II	Area III	Area IV	Area V	Area VI	Area VII	Area VIII
72 Asset assessment principles and methods	◆			◆			◆	◆
73 Capacity and needs assessment principles and methods	◆			◆			◆	◆
74 Health impact assessment principles and methods	◆			◆			◆	◆
75 Types of data (e.g., primary, secondary, qualitative, quantitative)	◆			◆			◆	◆
76 Data characteristics (e.g., reliability, validity, fairness, bias)	◆			◆				◆
77 Data collection methods (e.g., observation, survey, literature review, focus groups)	◆			◆	◆		◆	◆
78 Data collection instrumentation (e.g., authentic assessment, survey)	◆			◆				◆
79 Qualitative data analysis	◆			◆				◆
80 Quantitative data analysis	◆			◆				◆
81 Descriptive statistics	◆			◆			◆	◆

Section VI: Core Knowledge Items

Knowledge of: RESEARCH, EVALUATION, AND DATA COLLECTION	Area I Assessment of Needs and Capacity	Area II Planning	Area III Implementation	Area IV Evaluation and Research	Area V Advocacy	Area VI Communication	Area VII Leadership and Management	Area VIII Ethics and Professionalism
82 Inferential statistics	◆			◆			◆	◆
83 Levels of measurement (e.g., nominal, ordinal)	◆			◆				
84 Methods of reporting (e.g., graphs, infographics, charts, tables, narrative)	◆	◆		◆		◆	◆	◆
85 Identification and evaluation of databases for population data (e.g., census, CDC Wonder, BRFSS, YRBSS)	◆			◆				
86 Identification and evaluation of research and literature databases (e.g., MedLine)	◆			◆				
87 Epidemiology	◆			◆			◆	
88 Economic evaluation (e.g., cost analyses, return on investment)				◆			◆	◆
89 Value on investment				◆			◆	
90 Types of evaluation (e.g., process, impact, outcome, formative, summative)		◆	◆	◆	◆	◆	◆	◆
91 Evaluation models		◆	◆	◆	◆	◆	◆	◆
92 Program evaluation		◆	◆	◆	◆	◆	◆	◆
93 Health indicators	◆	◆						
94 Health Appraisals, Health Risk Assessment	◆			◆				◆
95 Evaluation of research studies and other professional literature				◆	◆		◆	◆
96 Research/evaluation design and methodology				◆	◆	◆		◆
97 Sampling principles and methods	◆			◆	◆	◆		◆

Section VI: Core Knowledge Items

Knowledge of: **RESEARCH, EVALUATION, AND DATA COLLECTION**	Assessment of Needs and Capacity **Area I**	Planning **Area II**	Implementation **Area III**	Evaluation and Research **Area IV**	Advocacy **Area V**	Communication **Area VI**	Leadership and Management **Area VII**	Ethics and Professionalism **Area VIII**
98 Institutional Review Board (IRB)	◆			◆				◆
99 Pilot testing principles and practices	◆	◆	◆	◆	◆	◆		◆
100 Considerations in the development of recommendations from evaluation and research findings	◆			◆	◆	◆	◆	◆
101 Dissemination of research/evaluation				◆				◆
102 Translation of research into practice				◆	◆	◆	◆	◆
103 Community-based participatory research	◆	◆		◆				◆
104 Quality improvement principles and methods			◆	◆			◆	◆
Knowledge of: **MANAGEMENT, BUDGET, ADMINISTRATION AND HUMAN RESOURCES**	**Area I**	**Area II**	**Area III**	**Area IV**	**Area V**	**Area VI**	**Area VII**	**Area VIII**
105 Budget development and forecasting							◆	◆
106 Budget management							◆	◆
107 Responding to requests for proposals, information, funding, quotes		◆					◆	◆
108 Solicitation and evaluation of proposals		◆					◆	◆
109 Creation, negotiation, and execution of contracts, including Memoranda of Understanding/Agreement							◆	◆
110 Leadership principles and models							◆	

Section VI: Core Knowledge Items

Knowledge of: MANAGEMENT, BUDGET, ADMINISTRATION AND HUMAN RESOURCES	Assessment of Needs and Capacity Area I	Planning Area II	Implementation Area III	Evaluation and Research Area IV	Advocacy Area V	Communication Area VI	Leadership and Management Area VII	Ethics and Professionalism Area VIII
111 Identification of funding sources (e.g., governmental, nongovernmental), proposal writing, and required reporting							◆	◆
112 Management theory, principles, and practices							◆	
113 Management, recruitment, retention, supervision, and evaluation of personnel, including paraprofessionals (e.g., community health workers, peer counselors, patient navigators, health coach)							◆	◆
114 Management, recruitment, retention, supervision, and evaluation of volunteers							◆	◆
115 Personality traits and group dynamics	◆	◆	◆		◆	◆	◆	
116 Management of other resources (e.g., equipment, facilities)							◆	◆
117 Stakeholder identification and relationship management	◆	◆		◆	◆		◆	
118 Team building and conflict resolution methods							◆	◆
119 Planning tools (e.g., timelines, Gantt charts)		◆	◆	◆			◆	
Knowledge of: COMMUNICATION	Area I	Area II	Area III	Area IV	Area V	Area VI	Area VII	Area VIII
120 Communication theories, models, principles, tools, and methods	◆	◆	◆		◆	◆	◆	
121 Assessment of materials			◆				◆	

Knowledge of: COMMUNICATION	Assessment of Needs and Capacity Area I	Planning Area II	Implementation Area III	Evaluation and Research Area IV	Advocacy Area V	Communication Area VI	Leadership and Management Area VII	Ethics and Professionalism Area VIII
122 Marketing principles and methods (e.g., persuasive communication)					◆	◆		
123 Social marketing					◆	◆		
124 Media literacy						◆		
125 Media relations						◆	◆	
126 Public relations						◆	◆	
127 Public speaking			◆		◆	◆	◆	
128 Social media tools and platforms use and management					◆	◆	◆	◆
129 Digital content development and management						◆	◆	
Knowledge of: ADVOCACY	Area I	Area II	Area III	Area IV	Area V	Area VI	Area VII	Area VIII
130 Administrative, legislative, regulatory, and judicial bodies and structure	◆	◆	◆		◆	◆	◆	
131 Civic responsibility (e.g., voter registration, run and/ or hold political office, attend community meetings)					◆		◆	
132 Organizational policy development and governance					◆		◆	
133 Advocacy terminology, principles, and methods					◆	◆		
134 Media advocacy					◆	◆		
Knowledge of: OTHER	Area I	Area II	Area III	Area IV	Area V	Area VI	Area VII	Area VIII
135 Foundational information about communicable diseases, non-communicable diseases, and injury prevention	◆	◆						◆

SECTION VI

Section VI: Core Knowledge Items

	Knowledge of: OTHER	Assessment of Needs and Capacity Area I	Planning Area II	Implementation Area III	Evaluation and Research Area IV	Advocacy Area V	Communication Area VI	Leadership and Management Area VII	Ethics and Professionalism Area VIII
136	Foundational information about dimensions of health and wellbeing (e.g., mental, social, physical, spiritual)	◆	◆						◆
137	Personal health behaviors	◆	◆						
138	Emergency preparedness and safety	◆	◆				◆	◆	
139	Environmental health	◆				◆		◆	◆
140	Mission and role of voluntary health organizations	◆	◆			◆		◆	
141	Global health	◆				◆			◆
142	Urban and rural health	◆				◆			◆
143	Levels of prevention (primary, secondary, tertiary)	◆	◆			◆		◆	
144	Current, social, and emerging technology	◆	◆	◆	◆	◆	◆	◆	◆
145	Emerging health issues	◆				◆			◆

Note. Knowledge item(s) link(s) to specific Area(s) of Responsibility are indicated by an asterisk (◆)

References

Airhihenbuwa, C. O., Cottrell, R. R., Adeyanju, M., Auld, M. E., Lysoby, L., & Smith, B. J. (2005). The National Health Educator Competencies Update Project: Celebrating a milestone and recommending next steps to the profession. *Health Education & Behavior, 32*(6), 722-724. https://doi.org/10.1177/1090198105282523

Allegrante, J. P., Airhihenbuwa, C. O., Auld, M. E., Birch, D. B., Roe, K. M., & Smith, B. J. (2004). Toward a unified system of accreditation for professional preparation in health education: Final report of the National Task Force on Accreditation in Health Education. *Health Education & Behavior, 31*(6), 1-16. https://doi.org/10.1080/19325037.2004.10604775

Allegrante, J. P., & Auld, M. E. (2019). Advancing the promise of digital technology and social media to promote population health. *Health Education & Behavior 46*(2s), 5-7. https://doi.org/10.1177/1090198119875929

Allegrante, J. P., Barry, M. M., Airhihenbuwa, C. O., Auld, M. E., Collins, J. L., Lamarre, M. C., Magnusson, G., McQueen, D.V., Mittlemark, M. B., & members of Galway Consensus Conference. (2009). Domains of core competency, standards, and quality assurance for building global capacity in health promotion: The Galway Consensus Conference Statement. *Health Education & Behavior, 36*(3), 476-82. https://doi.org/10.1177/1090198109333950

Allegrante, J. P., Barry, M. M., Auld, M. E., & Lamarre, M. C. (2012). Galway revisited: Tracking global progress in core competencies and quality assurance for health education and health promotion. *Health Education & Behavior, 39*(6), 643-647. https://doi org/10.1177/1090198112465089

American Educational Research Association, American Psychological Association, & National Council on Measurement in Education. (2014). *The standards for educational and psychological testing.*

Auld, M. E. (2017). Health education careers in a post-health reform era. *Health Promotion Practice, 18*(5), 629-635. https://doi.org/10.1177/1524839917726495

Bruening, R. A., Coronado, F., Auld, M. E., Benenson, G., & Simone, P. (2018). Health education workforce: Opportunities and challenges. *Preventing Chronic Disease, 15*(89), 1-3. https://doi.org/10.5888/pcd15.180045

Capwell, E., Cox, C., Taub, A., Auld, M., & Berhanu, E. (2019). Quality assurance in professional preparation of community/public health education specialists: Contributions of SABPAC. *Pedagogy in Health Promotion 5*(1), 62-69. https://doi.org/10.1177/2373379918756426

Chambliss, M. L., Lineberry, S. N., Evans, W. M., & Bibeau, D. L. (2014). Adding health education specialists to your practice. *Family Practice Management 21*(2), 10-15. https://www.aafp.org/fpm/2014/0300/p10.html

Chaney, B. H., Paravattil, B., Lysoby, L., Rehrig, M., Elmore, L., & Gambescia, S. F. (2013). A summative report of applications submitted for the Experience Documentation Opportunity (EDO) for the Master Certified Health Education Specialist Credential. *Health Promotion Practice, 14*(3), 354-363. https://doi.org/10.1177/1524839912455176

Cleary, H. P. (1995). *The credentialing of health educators: An historical account*, 1970-1990. National Commission for Health Education Credentialing, Inc.

Coalition of National Health Education Organizations. (2011). *Code of ethics for the health education profession*. http://www.cnheo.org/ethics-of-the-profession.html

Coalition of National Health Education Organizations. (2018). *Profession-wide strategic plan*. http://www.cnheo.org/PDF_files/CNHEO_Strategic_Plan.pdf

REFERENCES

References

Cottrell, R. R., Auld, M. E., Birch, D. A., Taub, A., King, L. R., & Allegrante, J. P. (2012). Progress and directions in professional credentialing for health education in the United States. *Health Education & Behavior*, *39*(6), 681-694. https://doi.org/10.1177/1090198112466096

Cottrell, R. R., Girvan, J. T., Seabert, D. M., Spear, C., McKenzie, J. F. (2018). *Principles and foundations of health promotion and education* (7th ed.). Pearson.

Cottrell, R .R., Lysoby, L., Rasar King, L., Airhihenbuwa, C. O., Roe, K. M., & Allegrante, J. P. (2009). Current developments in accreditation and certification for health promotion and health education: A perspective on systems of quality assurance in the United States. *Health Education & Behavior*, *36*(3), 451-463. https://doi.org/10.1177/1090198109333965

Council for the Accreditation of Educator Preparation (CAEP). (2015). *History of CAEP*. http://caepnet.org/about/history/

Council on Education for Public Health. (2005). *Accreditation criteria for public health programs*. https://ceph.org/about/org-info/criteria-procedures-documents/criteria-procedures/

Council on Education for Public Health. (2019a). *List of accredited schools and programs*. https://ceph.org/about/org-info/who-we-accredit/accredited/#programs

Council on Education for Public Health. (2019b). *List of Applicants*. https://ceph.org/about/org-info/who-we-accredit/applicants/

Dennis, D. L., & Mahoney, B. S. (2008). *The CHES examination: Standards and statistical information*. https://assets.speakcdn.com/assets/2251/spring2008bulletin.pdf

Dennis, D. L., McKenzie, J. F., & Chen, W. W. (2012). The value of CHES (and now MCHES)?-A commentary. *American Journal of Health Education*, *43*(3), 130-131.

Doyle, E. I., Caro, C. M., Lysoby, L., Auld, M. E., Smith, B., & Muenzen, P. (2012). The National Health Educator Job Analysis 2010: Process and outcomes. *Health Education & Behavior*, *39*(3), 695-708. https://doi.org/10.1177/1090198112463393

Durley, C. C. (2005, August 9). *The NOCA guide to understanding credentialing concepts*. National Organization for Competency Assurance. http://www.cvacert.org/documents/CredentialingConcepts-NOCA.pdf

Figueroa, J. L., Birch, D. A., King, L. R., & Cottrell, R. R. (2015). CEPH accreditation of stand-alone baccalaureate programs: A preliminary mapping exercise. *Health Promotion Practice*, *16*(1), 115-121. https://doi.org/10.1177/1524839914535778

Gilmore, G. D., Olsen, L. K., Taub, A., & Connell, D. (2005). Overview of the national health educator competencies update project 1998-2004. *Health Education & Behavior*, *32*(6), 725-737. https://doi.org/10.1080/19325037.2005.10608209

Institute for Credentialing Excellence. (2009). *National Commission for Certifying Agencies standards for accreditation of certification programs*.

Institute for Credentialing Excellence. (2014). *National Commission for Certifying Agencies standards for the accreditation of certification programs*.

Institute for Credentialing Excellence. (2016). *National Commission for Certifying Agencies standards for the accreditation of certification programs*.

Institute of Medicine. (2003). *Committee on Educating Public Health Professionals for the 21st Century* (K. Gebbie, L. Rosenstock, & L. M. Hernandez, Eds.). National Academies Press.

References

International Accreditation Service. (n.d.). *Personnel Certification Bodies*. ISO/IED Standard 17024. https://www.iasonline.org/services/personnel-certification-bodies/

International Organization for Standardization. (2012). *Conformity assessment – General requirements for bodies operating certification of persons* (ISO/IEC 17024:2012). https://www.iso.org/standard/52993.html

Joint Committee on Health Education and Promotion Terminology. (2012). Report of the 2011 joint committee on health education and promotion terminology. *American Journal of Health Education, 43*(2), SA, S1-S19.

Livingood, W. C., & Auld, M. E. (2001). The credentialing of a population-based profession: Lessons learned from health education certification. *Journal of Public Health Management and Practice, 7*(4), 38-45. https://doi.org/10.1097/00124784-200107040-00006

McKenzie, J. F., Dennis, D., Auld, M. E., Lysoby, L., Doyle, E., Muenzen, P. M., Caro, C. M., & Kusorgbor-Narh, C. S. (2016). Health education specialist practice analysis 2015 (HESPA 2015): Process and outcomes. *Health Education & Behavior, 43*(3), 286-295. https://doi.org/10.1177/1090198116639258

McKenzie, J. F., Neiger, B. L., Thackeray, R. (2017). *Planning, Implementing & Evaluating Health Promotion Programs* (7th ed.). Pearson.

National Commission for Health Education Credentialing, Inc. (1985). *A framework for the development of competency-based curricula for entry-level health educators.*

National Commission for Health Education Credentialing, Inc. (1996). *A competency-based framework for professional development of certified health education specialists.*

National Commission for Health Education Credentialing, Inc. (2007). *The health education specialist: A study guide for professional competence* (5th ed.).

National Commission for Health Education Credentialing, Inc. (2008). *CHES exam receives "Gold Standard" NCCA accreditation.* https://www.speakcdn.com/assets/2251/fall2008bulletin_reduced.pdf

National Commission for Health Education Credentialing, Inc. (2009). *An Advanced Level Credential.* https://www.speakcdn.com/assets/2251/fall_2009_bulletin.pdf

National Commission for Health Education Credentialing, Inc. (2019, April 1). *Continuing Competency. Policies and procedures for renewal and recertification manual*: Effective April 1, 2019. https://www.nchec.org/continuing-competency.

National Commission for Health Education Credentialing, Inc., American Association for Health Education, & Society for Public Health Education. (1999). *A competency based framework for graduate-level health educators.*

National Commission for Health Education Credentialing, Inc., Society for Public Health Education, & American Association for Health Education. (2006). *A competency-based framework for health educators – 2006.*

National Commission for Health Education Credentialing, Inc., Society for Public Health Education, & American Association for Health Education. (2010). *A competency-based framework for health education specialists – 2010.*

National Commission for Health Education Credentialing, Inc., & Society for Public Health Education. (2015). *A competency-based framework for health education specialists – 2015.*

References

Office of Management and Budget. (2000). *Standard occupational classification manual, 2000*. U.S. Government Printing Office.

Society for Public Health Education. Ad Hoc Task Force on Professional Preparation and Practice of Health Education. (1977). Guidelines for the preparation and practice of professional health educators. *Health Education Monographs, 5*(1), 75-89.

Society for Public Health Education, & American Association for Health Education. (1997). *Standards for the preparation of graduate-level health educators.*

Society for Public Health Education, & American Association for Health Education. (2007). *SOPHE/ AAHE baccalaureate program approval committee manual: Criteria, process, & procedures for quality assurance in community health education.*

Taub, A., Birch, D. A., Auld, M. E., Lysoby, L., & Rasar-King, L. (2009). Strengthening quality assurance in health education: Recent milestones and future directions. *Health Promotion Practice, 10*(2), 192-200. https://doi.org/10.1177/1524839908329854

Taub, A., Goekler, S., Auld, M. E., Birch, D. A., Mueller, S., Wengert, D., & Allegrante, J. (2014). Accreditation of professional preparation programs for school health educators: The changing landscape. *Health Education & Behavior, 41*(4), 349 – 58. https://doi.org/10.1177/1090198114539686

Teacher Education Accreditation Council (TEAC). (2014). https://www.chea.org/teacher-education-accreditation-council

United States Department of Health, Education and Welfare, Health Resources Administration, Bureau of Health Manpower. (1978). *Preparation and practice of community, patient, and school health educators: Proceedings of the workshop on commonalities and differences*. Division of Allied Health Professions.

United States Department of Labor, Bureau of Labor Statistics. (2018). 21-1091 *Health education specialists and 21-1094 community health workers*. 2018 Standard Occupational Classification System. https://www.bls.gov/soc/2018/major_groups.htm#21-0000

Wilson, K. L., Dennis, D. L., Gambescia, S. F., Chen, W. W., & Lysoby, L. (2012). Using an experience documentation opportunity to certify advanced-level health education specialists. *Health Education & Behavior, 39*(6), 709-718. https://doi.org/10.1177/1090198112465621

REFERENCES

Appendix A: Glossary

The glossary is presented to explain terms used in this publication. These definitions are not all inclusive, but are intended to convey the meaning of terms within the context of this document.

Advanced 1-level - The practice level of a health education specialist with a minimum of a baccalaureate degree with professional preparation in the field of health education plus various combinations of degree (baccalaureate or master's) and years of experience.

Advanced 2-level - The practice level of a health education specialist with a minimum of a doctoral degree in the field of health education, irrespective of years of experience.

Area of Responsibility - The major categories of performance expectations of a proficient health education specialist.

Certified Health Education Specialist (CHES®) - "An individual who has met required academic preparation qualifications, successfully passed a competency-based examination administered by the National Commission for Health Education Credentialing, Inc., and who satisfies the continuing education requirement to maintain the national credential" (Joint Committee on Health Education and Promotion Terminology, 2012, p. 8).

Master Certified Health Education Specialist (MCHES®) - "An advanced-level practitioner who has met required academic preparation qualifications, worked in the field for a minimum of five years, has successfully passed a competency-based assessment administered by the National Commission for Health Education Credentialing, Inc., and who satisfies the continuing education requirement to maintain the national credential" (Joint Committee on Health Education and Promotion Terminology, 2012, p. 8-9).

Certification (professional) - "The voluntary process by which a non-governmental entity grants a time-limited recognition and use of a credential to an individual after verifying that he or she has met predetermined and standardized criteria. It is the vehicle that a profession or occupation uses to differentiate among its members, using standards, sometimes developed through a consensus driven process, based on existing legal and psychometric requirements" (Durley, 2005, p. 5).

Credentialing - An umbrella term for the process by which an entity, authorized and qualified to do so, grants formal recognition (i.e., accreditation, licensure, registration, certification) to or records the recognition status of individuals, organizations, institutions, programs, processes, services, or products that meet predetermined and standardized criteria (Durley 2005, p. 5).

Coalition - An alliance, often temporary, that allows two or more groups or organizations to promote a common cause (AAHE, NCHEC, & SOPHE, 1999).

Competency - A broadly defined skill or ability necessary for successful performance as a health education specialist. A Competency defines an activity that elaborates on an Area of Responsibility. The set of Competencies for an Area of Responsibility offers a comprehensive and detailed description of the Area of Responsibility.

Entry-level - The practice level of a health education specialist with a minimum of a baccalaureate degree in the field of health education who has yet to obtain extensive work experience.

Appendix A: Glossary

Health advocacy - "The process by which the actions of individuals or groups attempt to bring social, environmental and/or organizational change on behalf of a particular health goal, program, interest or population" (Joint Committee on Health Education and Promotion Terminology, 2012, p. 12).

Health education - "Any combination of planned learning experiences using evidence-based practices and/or sound theories that provide the opportunity to acquire knowledge, attitudes, and skills needed to adopt and maintain healthy behaviors" (Joint Committee on Health Education and Promotion Terminology, 2012, p. 12).

Health education profession - "A profession that uses evidence-based practice, and behavioral and organizational change principles to develop, plan, implement, and evaluate interventions that enable individuals, groups, and communities to achieve personal, environmental, and societal health" (Joint Committee on Health Education and Promotion Terminology, 2012, p. 12).

Health education specialist - "An individual who has met, at a minimum, baccalaureate-level required academic preparation qualifications, who serves in a variety of settings, and is able to use appropriate educational strategies and methods to facilitate the development of policies, procedures, interventions, and systems conducive to the health of individuals, groups, and communities" (Joint Committee on Health Education and Promotion Terminology, 2012, p. 13).

Health literacy - "The degree to which individuals have the capacity to obtain, interpret, and understand basic health information and services and the competence to make appropriate health decisions" (Joint Committee on Health Education and Promotion Terminology, 2012, p. 13).

Health promotion - "Any planned combination of educational, political, environmental, regulatory, or organizational mechanisms that support actions and conditions of living that are conducive to the health of individuals, groups, and communities" (Joint Committee on Health Education and Promotion Terminology, 2012, p. 14).

Knowledge Items - The validated list of statements required for proficient performance as a health education specialist.

Professional development - "Education and training to maintain and enhance one's competence in health education and health promotion following a previously attained level of professional preparation" (Joint Committee on Health Education and Promotion Terminology, 2012, p. 14).

Professional preparation - "An undergraduate or graduate course of study based on the Areas of Responsibility, Competencies, and Sub-competencies for health education offered through an accredited college or university, that is designed to prepare individuals to practice competently in health education" (Joint Committee on Health Education and Promotion Terminology, 2012, p. 14).

Standard - The predetermined level of performance at which a criterion will be considered met. If a desired condition or characteristic (e.g., curricular content that assures development of specific health education Competencies) is the criterion, the standard then expresses the minimum acceptable content that will satisfy the expectation (NCHEC, AAHE & SOPHE, 1999, p. 60).

Sub-competency - A cluster of simpler but essential related skills or abilities within a Competency. The set of Sub-competencies clarifies the expectations for health education specialists at the baccalaureate, master's, and doctoral level.

Appendix B: Comparison of the Sub-competencies of the HESPA I 2015 Model and the HESPA II 2020 Model

The HESPA II 2020 Model reflects the contemporary practice of health education specialists at the entry-, advanced 1-, and advanced 2- levels. The updated model differs from the HESPA I 2015 model. It now contains Eight Areas of Responsibility, a consolidation of related Competencies and Sub-competencies from the HESPA I 2015 Model, and the addition of some new Sub-competencies. Seasoned health education specialists may also note slight wording changes to help convey the nuances of health education practice (see Section V for a detailed explanation of the changes). The HESPA II 2020 Model serves as the framework for certification, professional preparation, and professional development. Thus, health education specialists may need to adapt the criteria and materials used for these three purposes so as to align with the updated model. To help facilitate these adaptations, the coordinator of the NCHEC Division Board for Certification of Health Education Specialists led a volunteer group experienced in the use of the Framework to compare the Sub-Competencies structured within the Competencies and Areas of Responsibility of the HESPA I 2015 Model to the HESPA II 2020 Model. Tables B.1 and B.2 illustrate the results of this comparison: Table B.1 starts with the HESPA I 2015 Model (old) and Table B.2 starts with the new HESPA II 2020 Model (new). The comparison tables were completed with the intent to direct users to similar or related Sub-competencies that may be useful in making the transition from the HESPA I 2015 Model to the HESPA II 2020 Model. There is not a one-to-one correspondence between the HESPA I 2015 and HESPA II 2020 Sub-competencies. Also, some wording of Sub-competencies has changed. Therefore, users are urged to carefully consider the wording of the given Sub-competency and make their own determination as to whether the statement(s) are applicable.

Table B.1 can be used to identify specific Sub-competencies in the HESPA I 2015 Model that were retained, re-assigned, and/or revised and integrated within a different Area of Responsibility, Competency or Sub-competency in the HESPA II 2020 Model. For example, the first Sub-competency in the HESPA I 2015 Model under Area of Responsibility I was *1.1.1 Define the priority population to be assessed.* Slightly different wording with similar intent appears in the HESPA II 2020 Model renumbered as Sub-competency *1.1.2 identify priority population(s).* Another example is HESPA I 2015 Model, Sub-competency *7.4.10 Develop materials that contribute to the professional literature* which was reassigned to Area of Responsibility VIII with similar wording in Sub-competency *8.4.6 Develop presentations and publications that contribute to the professional literature.*

Entries in the table with the same wording are identified by "same wording" in the right hand column under comments. For example, in the HESPA I 2015 Model, Sub-competency *1.2.2 Establish collaborative relationships and agreements that facilitate access* to data remains the same under HESPA II 2020 as Sub-competency *1.2.2 Establish collaborative relationships and agreements that facilitate access to data.* Another example is HESPA I 2015 Model Sub-competency *1.7.3 Prioritize health education/promotion needs* is the same wording as HESPA II 2020 Model Sub-competency *1.4.2 Prioritize health education and promotion needs.*

If no apparent match was found, the words "no match" appear in the right hand column. HESPA I 2015 Model Sub-competency *1.4.3 Summarize the capacity of priority populations to meet the needs of the priority populations* is an example of a Sub-competency with no match. Though the comparison results are useful for the realignment of items on the certification exam and for adjusting curricula in professional preparation programs, the comparison was based on specific

Appendix B: Comparison of the Sub-competencies of the HESPA I 2015 Model and the HESPA II 2020 Model

wording, not on intent of use. Users must carefully examine the intent of use of the Competency or Sub-competency when considering the information presented in Tables B.1 and B.2.

The levels (entry, advanced-1, and advanced-2) are indicated by symbols. The entry-level Sub-competencies have no symbol, the advanced-1 level (▲), and the advanced-2 level (■). As indicated in Table B.1, some Sub-competencies in the HESPA I 2015 Model may now be in a different level of practice in the HESPA II 2020 Model. For example, in the HESPA I 2015 Model, entry-level Sub-competency *1.3.4 Train personnel assisting with data collection* is now reflected in the HESPA II 2020 Model as Sub-competency *4.3.1 Train data collectors* at the advanced-2 level (■). Users are reminded that this Model is hierarchical, meaning the advanced-levels build on the previous level. Therefore, the entry-level Sub-competencies apply to all levels. The advanced 2-level would also include advanced 1-level Sub-competencies.

The format of Table B.2 is similar to that of Table B.1. However, Table B.2 contains the Areas of Responsibility, Competencies, and Sub-competencies of the HESPA II 2020 Model. The right hand column indicates similarly worded Competencies or Sub-competencies in the HESPA I 2015 Model. For some, "no match" is listed in the comments column to denote that no Competency or Sub-competency containing that specific wording existed in the HESPA I 2015 Model. The same caution provided for interpreting the words "no match" in Table B.1 should also be used in interpreting "no match" in Table B.2. It should be noted that the comparison was based on specific wording, not on intent of use. It is up to users to carefully examine the intent of use of the Sub-competency when considering the information presented in Tables B.1 and B.2.

The HESPA II 2020 Model shows the consolidation of some of the Competencies and Sub-competencies of the HESPA I 2015 Model, along with the addition of components and updated wording. The consolidation and revised wording have resulted in decreased redundancy and increased differentiation of the Sub-competencies. The changes also reflect the contemporary practice of health education specialists at the entry-, advanced 1-, and advanced 2-levels.

Appendix B.1: Comparison of the Competencies and Sub-competencies of the HESPA I 2015 Model to the HESPA II 2020 Model

Table: B.1
Comparison of the Competencies and Sub-competencies of the HESPA I 2015 Model (Old) to the HESPA II 2020 Model (New)

Many of the HESPA 2015 Sub-competencies correlate to similar HESPA II 2020 Sub-competencies. If the Sub-competency is worded the same in both Frameworks, it is indicated under comments. All advanced-1 Sub-competencies are indicated by the symbol (▲), and the advanced-2 Sub-competencies are indicated by the symbol (■). "No match" indicated no direct/similar Sub-competency.

Key: Entry level = No symbol; Advanced-1 (▲); Advanced-2 (■)
Sub-competency worded the same in both Frameworks is indicated under comments

HESPA I Code	HESPA I 2015	HESPA II Code	HESPA II 2020	Comments
	Area I: Assess Needs, Resources, and Capacity for Health Education/Promotion			
1.1	**Plan assessment process for health education/promotion**			
1.1.1	Define the priority population to be assessed	1.1.2	Identify priority population(s)	
1.1.2	Identify existing and necessary resources to conduct assessments	1.1.3	Identify existing and available resources, policies, programs, practices, and interventions	
1.1.3	Engage priority populations, partners, and stakeholders to participate in the assessment process	1.1.5	Recruit and/or engage priority population(s), partners, and stakeholders to participate throughout all steps in the assessment, planning, implementation, and evaluation processes	
1.1.4 ▲	Apply theories and/or models to assessment process	8.1.5	Use evidence-informed theories, models, and strategies	
1.1.5	Apply ethical principles to the assessment process	8.1.1	Apply professional codes of ethics and ethical principles throughout assessment, planning, implementation, evaluation and research, communication, consulting, and advocacy processes	

Appendix B.1: Comparison of the Competencies and Sub-competencies of the HESPA I 2015 Model to the HESPA II 2020 Model

Key: Entry level = No symbol; Advanced-1 (▲); Advanced-2 (■)
   Sub-competency worded the same in both Frameworks is indicated under comments

HESPA I Code	HESPA I 2015	HESPA II Code	HESPA II 2020	Comments
	Area I: Assess Needs, Resources, and Capacity for Health Education/Promotion			**Comments**
1.2	**Access existing information and data related to health**			
1.2.1	Identify sources of secondary data related to health	1.2.1	Identify primary data, secondary data, and evidence-informed resources	
1.2.2 ▲	Establish collaborative relationships and agreements that facilitate access to data	1.2.2 ▲	Establish collaborative relationships and agreements that facilitate access to data	Same wording
1.2.3	Review related literature	1.2.3	Conduct a literature review.	
1.2.4	Identify gaps in the secondary data	1.2.6	Identify data gaps	
1.2.5	Extract data from existing databases	1.2.4	Procure secondary data	
1.2.6	Determine the validity of existing data	1.2.5	Determine the validity and reliability of the secondary data	
1.3	**Collect primary data to determine needs**			
1.3.1	Identify data collection instruments	1.2.7	Determine primary data collection needs, instruments, methods, and procedures	
1.3.2	Select data collection methods for use in assessment	1.2.7	Determine primary data collection needs, instruments, methods, and procedures	
1.3.3	Develop data collection procedures	1.2.7	Determine primary data collection needs, instruments, methods, and procedures	
1.3.4	Train personnel assisting with data collection	4.3.1 ■	Train data collectors	
1.3.5	Implement quantitative and/or qualitative data collection	1.2.8 / 4.3.2	Adhere to established procedures to collect data / Implement data collection procedures	

Appendix B.1: Comparison of the Competencies and Sub-competencies of the HESPA I 2015 Model to the HESPA II 2020 Model

Key: Entry level = No symbol; Advanced-1 (▲); Advanced-2 (■)
   Sub-competency worded the same in both Frameworks is indicated under comments

HESPA I Code	HESPA I 2015	HESPA II Code	HESPA II 2020	Comments
	Area I: Assess Needs, Resources, and Capacity for Health Education/Promotion			
1.4	**Analyze relationships among behavioral, environmental, and other factors that influence health**			
1.4.1	Identify and analyze factors that influence health behaviors	1.3.2 / 1.3.3	Determine the knowledge, attitudes, beliefs, skills, and behaviors that impact the health and health literacy of the priority population(s) / Identify the social, cultural, economic, political, and environmental factors that impact the health and/or learning processes of the priority population(s)	
1.4.2	Identify and analyze factors that impact health	1.3.2 / 1.3.3	Determine the knowledge, attitudes, beliefs, skills, and behaviors that impact the health and health literacy of the priority population(s) / Identify the social, cultural, economic, political, and environmental factors that impact the health and/or learning processes of the priority population(s)	
1.4.3	Identify the impact of emerging social, economic, and other trends on health	1.3.3 / 5.1.1	Identify the social, cultural, economic, political, and environmental factors that impact the health and/or learning processes of the priority population(s) / Examine the determinants of health and their underlying causes (e.g., poverty, trauma, and population-based discrimination) related to identified health issues	
1.5	**Examine factors that influence the process by which people learn**			
1.5.1	Identify and analyze factors that foster or hinder the learning process	1.3.3	Identify the social, cultural, economic, political, and environmental factors that impact the health and/or learning processes of the priority population(s)	

Appendix B.1: Comparison of the Competencies and Sub-competencies of the HESPA I 2015 Model to the HESPA II 2020 Model

Key: Entry level = No symbol; Advanced-1 (▲); Advanced-2 (■)
Sub-competency worded the same in both Frameworks is indicated under comments

HESPA I Code	HESPA I 2015	HESPA II Code	HESPA II 2020	
	Area I: Assess Needs, Resources, and Capacity for Health Education/Promotion			**Comments**
1.5.2	Identify and analyze factors that foster or hinder knowledge acquisition	1.3.2	Determine the knowledge, attitudes, beliefs, skills, and behaviors that impact the health and health literacy of the priority population(s)	
		1.3.3	Identify the social, cultural, economic, political, and environmental factors that impact the health and/or learning processes of the priority population(s)	
1.5.3	Identify and analyze factors that influence attitudes and beliefs	1.3.2	Determine the knowledge, attitudes, beliefs, skills, and behaviors that impact the health and health literacy of the priority population(s)	
1.5.4	Identify and analyze factors that foster or hinder acquisition of skills	1.3.2	Determine the knowledge, attitudes, beliefs, skills, and behaviors that impact the health and health literacy of the priority population(s)	
		1.3.3	Identify the social, cultural, economic, political, and environmental factors that impact the health and/or learning processes of the priority population(s)	
1.6	**Examine factors that enhance or impede the process of health education/promotion**			
1.6.1	Determine the extent of available health education/promotion programs and interventions	1.3.4	Assess existing and available resources, policies, programs, practices, and interventions	
		1.3.5	Determine the capacity (available resources, policies, programs, practices, and interventions) to improve and/or maintain health	
1.6.2	Identify policies related to health education/promotion	1.3.4	Assess existing and available resources, policies, programs, practices, and interventions	
		1.3.5	Determine the capacity (available resources, policies, programs, practices, and interventions) to improve and/or maintain health	

Appendix B.1: Comparison of the Competencies and Sub-competencies of the HESPA I 2015 Model to the HESPA II 2020 Model

Key: Entry level = No symbol; Advanced-1 (▲); Advanced-2 (■)
    Sub-competency worded the same in both Frameworks is indicated under comments

HESPA I Code	HESPA I 2015	HESPA II Code	HESPA II 2020	
	Area I: Assess Needs, Resources, and Capacity for Health Education/Promotion			**Comments**
1.6.3	Assess the effectiveness of existing health education/promotion programs and interventions	1.3.4	Assess existing and available resources, policies, programs, practices, and interventions	
1.6.4	Assess social, environmental, political, and other factors that may impact health education/promotion	1.1.4	Examine the factors and determinants that influence the assessment process	
		1.3.3	Identify the social, cultural, economic, political, and environmental factors that impact the health and/or learning processes of the priority population(s)	
		6.2.3	Identify factors that facilitate and/or hinder the intended outcome of the communication	
1.6.5	Analyze the capacity for providing necessary health education/promotion	1.3.5	Determine the capacity (available resources, policies, programs, practices, and interventions) to improve and/or maintain health	
1.7	**Determine needs for health education/promotion based on assessment findings**			
1.7.1 ▲	Synthesize assessment findings	1.4.1 ▲	Compare findings to norms, existing data, and other information	
		1.3.6	List the needs of the priority population(s)	
1.7.2	Identify current needs, resources, and capacity	1.3.6	List the needs of the priority population(s)	
		1.3.5	Determine the capacity (available resources, policies, programs, practices, and interventions) to improve and/or maintain health	
1.7.3	Prioritize health education/promotion needs	1.4.2	Prioritize health education and promotion needs	Same wording
1.7.4	Develop recommendations for health education/promotion based on assessment findings	1.4.4	Develop recommendations based on findings	
1.7.5	Report assessment findings	1.4.5	Report assessment findings	Same Wording

Appendix B.1: Comparison of the Competencies and Sub-competencies of the HESPA I 2015 Model to the HESPA II 2020 Model

Key: Entry level = No symbol; Advanced-1 (▲); Advanced-2 (■)

Sub-competency worded the same in both Frameworks is indicated under comments

HESPA I Code	HESPA I 2015	HESPA II Code	HESPA II 2020	
	Area II: Plan Health Education/ Promotion			**Comments**
2.1	**Involve priority populations, partners, and other stakeholders in the planning process**			
2.1.1	Identify priority populations, partners, and other stakeholders	1.1.2 5.1.5 7.1.1	Identify priority population(s) Identify existing coalition(s) or stakeholders that can be engaged in advocacy efforts Identify potential partners and stakeholders	
2.1.2	Use strategies to convene priority populations, partners, and other stakeholders	2.1.1 7.1.3	Convene priority populations, partners, and stakeholders Involve partners and stakeholders throughout the health education and promotion process in meaningful and sustainable ways	
2.1.3	Facilitate collaborative efforts among priority populations, partners, and other stakeholders	2.1.2	Facilitate collaborative efforts among priority populations, partners, and stakeholders	Same wording
2.1.4	Elicit input about the plan	2.2.2	Elicit input from priority populations, partners, and stakeholders regarding desired outcomes	
2.1.5	Obtain commitments to participate in health education/promotion	7.1.4 ▲	Execute formal and informal agreements with partners and stakeholders	
2.2	**Develop goals and objectives**			
2.2.1	Identify desired outcomes using the needs assessment results	2.2.1	Identify desired outcomes using the needs and capacity assessment	
2.2.2	Develop vision statement	2.2.3	Develop vision, mission, and goal statements for the intervention(s)	
2.2.3	Develop mission statement	2.2.3	Develop vision, mission, and goal statements for the intervention(s)	
2.2.4	Develop goal statements	2.2.3	Develop vision, mission, and goal statements for the intervention(s)	

APPENDIX B1

Appendix B.1: Comparison of the Competencies and Sub-competencies of the HESPA I 2015 Model to the HESPA II 2020 Model

Key: Entry level = No symbol; Advanced-1 (▲); Advanced-2 (■)
　　Sub-competency worded the same in both Frameworks is indicated under comments

HESPA I Code	HESPA I 2015	HESPA II Code	HESPA II 2020	Comments
	Area II: Planning			**Comments**
2.2.5	Develop specific, measurable, attainable, realistic, and time-sensitive objectives	2.2.4	Develop specific, measurable, achievable, realistic, and time-bound (SMART) objectives	
		5.1.4	Write specific, measurable, achievable, realistic, and time-bound (SMART) advocacy objective(s)	
		6.2.2	Write specific, measurable, achievable, realistic, and time-bound (SMART) communication objective(s)	
2.3	**Select or design strategies/ interventions**			
2.3.1 ▲	Select planning model(s) for health education/promotion	2.3.1	Select planning model(s) for health education and promotion	Same Wording
2.3.2 ▲	Assess efficacy of various strategies/ interventions to ensure consistency with objectives	2.3.3 ▲	Assess the effectiveness and alignment of existing interventions to desired outcomes	
2.3.3 ▲	Apply principles of evidence-based practice in selecting and/or designing strategies/interventions	8.1.5	Use evidence-informed theories, models, and strategies	
2.3.4	Apply principles of cultural competence in selecting and/or designing strategies/ interventions	2.3.4	Adopt, adapt, and/or develop tailored intervention(s) for priority population(s) to achieve desired outcomes	
		8.1.6	Apply principles of cultural humility, inclusion, and diversity in all aspects of practice (e.g., Culturally and Linguistically Appropriate Services (CLAS) standards and culturally responsive pedagogy)	
2.3.5	Address diversity within priority populations in selecting and/or designing strategies/interventions	2.3.4	Adopt, adapt, and/or develop tailored intervention(s) for priority population(s) to achieve desired outcomes	
		8.1.6	Apply principles of cultural humility, inclusion, and diversity in all aspects of practice (e.g., Culturally and Linguistically Appropriate Services (CLAS) standards and culturally responsive pedagogy)	
2.3.6	Identify delivery methods and settings to facilitate learning	1.3.3	Identify the social, cultural, economic, political, and environmental factors that impact the health and/or learning processes of the priority population(s)	

APPENDIX B1

Appendix B.1: Comparison of the Competencies and Sub-competencies of the HESPA I 2015 Model to the HESPA II 2020 Model

Key: Entry level = No symbol; Advanced-1 (▲); Advanced-2 (■)

Sub-competency worded the same in both Frameworks is indicated under comments

HESPA I Code	HESPA I 2015	HESPA II Code	HESPA II 2020		Comments
	Area II: Planning				**Comments**
2.3.7	Tailor strategies/interventions for priority populations	2.3.4	Adopt, adapt, and/or develop tailored intervention(s) for priority population(s) to achieve desired outcomes		
2.3.8	Adapt existing strategies/interventions as needed	2.3.4	Adopt, adapt, and/or develop tailored intervention(s) for priority population(s) to achieve desired outcomes		
2.3.9 ▲	Conduct pilot test of strategies/interventions	2.3.6 ▲	Conduct a pilot test of intervention(s)		
2.3.10 ▲	Refine strategies/interventions based on pilot feedback	2.3.7 ▲	Revise intervention(s) based on pilot feedback		
2.3.11	Apply ethical principles in selecting strategies and designing interventions	8.1.1	Apply professional codes of ethics and ethical principles throughout assessment, planning, implementation, evaluation and research, communication, consulting, and advocacy processes		
2.3.12	Comply with legal standards in selecting strategies and designing interventions	8.1.3	Comply with legal standards and regulatory guidelines in assessment, planning, implementation, evaluation and research, advocacy, management, communication, and reporting processes		
2.4	**Develop a plan for delivery of health/education promotion**				
2.4.1	Use theories and/or models to guide the delivery plan	2.3.2 ▲ 8.1.5	Create a logic model Use evidence-informed theories, models, and strategies		
2.4.2	Identify the resources involved in the delivery of health education/promotion	2.3.5 ▲	Plan for acquisition of required tools and resources		
2.4.3	Organize health education/promotion into a logical sequence	2.3.2 ▲ 2.4.1 ▲	Create a logic model Develop an implementation plan inclusive of logic model, work plan, responsible parties, timeline, marketing, and communication		
2.4.4	Develop a timeline for the delivery of health education/promotion	2.4.1 ▲	Develop an implementation plan inclusive of logic model, work plan, responsible parties, timeline, marketing, and communication		

Appendix B.1: Comparison of the Competencies and Sub-competencies of the HESPA I 2015 Model to the HESPA II 2020 Model

Key: Entry level = No symbol; Advanced-1 (▲); Advanced-2 (■)
  Sub-competency worded the same in both Frameworks is indicated under comments

HESPA I Code	HESPA I 2015	HESPA II Code	HESPA II 2020	Comments
	Area II: Planning			**Comments**
2.4.5	Develop marketing plan to deliver health program	2.4.2	Develop materials needed for implementation	
2.4.6	Select methods and/or channels for reaching priority populations	6.1.3	Identify communication channels (e.g., social media and mass media) available to and used by the audience(s)	
2.4.7	Analyze the opportunity for integrating health education/promotion into other programs	2.4.5 ▲	Plan for sustainability	
2.4.8 ▲	Develop a process for integrating health education/promotion into other programs when needed	2.4.5 ▲	Plan for sustainability	
2.4.9	Assess the sustainability of the delivery plan	2.4.5 ▲	Plan for sustainability	
2.4.10	Design and conduct pilot study of health education/promotion plan	2.3.6 ▲	Conduct a pilot test of intervention(s)	
2.5	**Address factors that influence implementation of health education/promotion**			
2.5.1	Identify and analyze factors that foster or hinder implementation	2.4.3 ▲	Address factors that influence implementation	
2.5.2	Develop plans and processes to overcome potential barriers to the implementation process	2.4.3 ▲	Address factors that influence implementation	
	Area III: Implement Health Education/Promotion			**Comments**
3.1	**Coordinate logistics necessary to implement plan**			
3.1.1	Create an environment conducive to learning	3.2.1	Create an environment conducive to learning	Same wording

APPENDIX B1

Appendix B.1: Comparison of the Competencies and Sub-competencies of the HESPA I 2015 Model to the HESPA II 2020 Model

Key: Entry level = No symbol; Advanced-1 (▲); Advanced-2 (■)
Sub-competency worded the same in both Frameworks is indicated under comments

HESPA I Code	HESPA I 2015	HESPA II Code	HESPA II 2020		Comments
	Area III: Implement Health Education/Promotion				**Comments**
3.1.2	Develop materials to implement plan	2.4.2	Develop materials needed for implementation		
3.1.3	Secure resources to implement plan	3.1.1	Secure implementation resources		
3.1.4	Arrange for needed services to implement plan	3.1.2 2.3.5 ▲	Arrange for implementation services Plan for acquisition of required tools and resources		
3.1.5	Apply ethical principles to the implemetation process	8.1.1	Apply professional codes of ethics and ethical principles throughout assessment, planning, implementation, evaluation and research, communication, consulting, and advocacy processes		
3.1.6	Comply with legal standards that apply to implementation	3.1.3 8.1.3	Comply with contractual obligations Comply with legal standards and regulatory guidelines in assessment, planning, implementation, evaluation and research, advocacy, management, communication, and reporting processes		
3.2	**Train staff members and volunteers involved in implementation of health education/promotion**				
3.2.1 ▲	Develop training objectives	3.1.4 ▲ 2.2.4	Establish training protocol Develop specific, measurable, achievable, realistic, and time-bound (SMART) objectives		
3.2.2	Recruit individuals needed in implementation	1.1.5 7.2.2	Recruit and/or engage priority population(s), partners, and stakeholders to participate throughout all steps in the assessment, planning, implementation, and evaluation processes Recruit individuals needed in implementation		Same wording
3.2.3 ▲	Identify training needs of individuals involved in implementation	7.2.3 ▲	Assess training needs		

APPENDIX B1

Appendix B.1: Comparison of the Competencies and Sub-competencies of the HESPA I 2015 Model to the HESPA II 2020 Model

Key: Entry level = No symbol; Advanced-1 (▲); Advanced-2 (■)
  Sub-competency worded the same in both Frameworks is indicated under comments

HESPA I Code	HESPA I 2015	HESPA II Code	HESPA II 2020	
	Area III: Implement Health Education/Promotion			**Comments**
3.2.4 ▲	Develop training using best practices	8.1.5	Use evidence-informed theories, models, and strategies	
		7.2.4 ▲	Plan training, including technical assistance and support	
		3.1.4 ▲	Establish training protocol	
3.2.5 ▲	Implement training	7.2.5 ▲	Implement training	Same wording
		3.1.5	Train staff and volunteers to ensure fidelity	
3.2.6 ▲	Provide support and technical assistance to those implementing the plan	7.2.4 ▲	Plan training, including technical assistance and support	
3.2.7 ▲	Evaluate training	7.2.6 ▲	Evaluate training as appropriate throughout the process	
3.2.8 ▲	Use evaluation findings to plan/modify future training	4.5.3 ■	Identify recommendations for quality improvement	
3.3	**Implement health education/ promotion plan**			
3.3.1	Collect baseline data	3.2.2	Collect baseline data	Same wording
3.3.2 ▲	Apply theories and/or models of implementation	8.1.5	Use evidence-informed theories, models, and strategies	
3.3.3	Assess readiness for implementation	2.4.3	Address factors that influence implementation	
3.3.4	Apply principles of diversity and cultural competence in implementing health education/promotion plan	8.1.6	Apply principles of cultural humility, inclusion, and diversity in all aspects of practice (e.g., Culturally and Linguistically Appropriate Services (CLAS) standards and culturally responsive pedagogy)	
		7.2.1	Develop culturally responsive content	
		7.3.1 ▲	Facilitate understanding and sensitivity for various cultures, values, and traditions	
3.3.5	Implement marketing plan	3.2.3	Implement a marketing plan	Same wording

Appendix B.1: Comparison of the Competencies and Sub-competencies of the HESPA I 2015 Model to the HESPA II 2020 Model

Key: Entry level = No symbol; Advanced-1 (▲); Advanced-2 (■)
Sub-competency worded the same in both Frameworks is indicated under comments

HESPA I Code	HESPA I 2015	HESPA II Code	HESPA II 2020	Comments
	Area III: Implement Health Education/Promotion			**Comments**
3.3.6	Deliver health education/promotion as designed	3.2.4	Deliver health education and promotion as designed	Same wording
3.3.7	Use a variety of strategies to deliver plan	3.2.5	Employ an appropriate variety of instructional methodologies	
3.4	**Monitor implementation of health education/promotion**			
3.4.1	Monitor progress in accordance with timeline	3.3.1	Monitor progress in accordance with the timeline	Same wording
3.4.2	Assess progress in achieving objectives	3.3.2	Assess progress in achieving objectives	Same wording
3.4.3	Ensure plan is implemented consistently	3.3.4	Ensure plan is implemented with fidelity	
3.4.4	Modify plan when needed	3.3.3	Modify interventions as needed to meet individual needs	
3.4.5	Monitor use of resources	3.3.5	Monitor use of resources	Same wording
3.4.6	Evaluate sustainability of implementation	3.3.6	Evaluate the sustainability of implementation	Same wording
3.4.7	Ensure compliance with legal standards	8.1.3	Comply with legal standards and regulatory guidelines in assessment, planning, implementation, evaluation and research, advocacy, management, communication, and reporting processes	
3.4.8	Monitor adherence to ethical principles in the implementation of health education/promotion	8.1.1	Apply professional codes of ethics and ethical principles throughout assessment, planning, implementation, evaluation and research, communication, consulting, and advocacy processes	

Appendix B.1: Comparison of the Competencies and Sub-competencies of the HESPA I 2015 Model to the HESPA II 2020 Model

Key: Entry level = No symbol; Advanced-1 (▲); Advanced-2 (■)

Sub-competency worded the same in both Frameworks is indicated under comments

HESPA I Code	HESPA I 2015	HESPA II Code	HESPA II 2020	Comments
	Area IV: Conduct Evaluation and Research Related to Health Education/Promotion			
4.1	**Develop evaluation plan for health education/promotion**			
4.1.1 ▲	Determine the purpose and goals of evaluation	4.1.1 ▲	Align the evaluation plan with the intervention goals and objectives	
4.1.2 ▲	Develop questions to be answered by the evaluation	4.1.5 ▲	Select an evaluation design model and the types of data to be collected	
4.1.3 ▲	Create a logic model to guide the evaluation process	4.1.3	Use a logic model and/or theory for evaluations	
4.1.4 ▲	Adapt/modify a logic model to guide the evaluation process	4.1.3 ▲	Use a logic model and/or theory for evaluations	
4.1.5 ▲	Assess needed and available resources to conduct evaluation	4.1.4 ▲	Assess capacity to conduct evaluation	
4.1.6 ▲	Determine the types of data (for example, qualitative, quantitative) to be collected	4.1.5 ▲	Select an evaluation design model and the types of data to be collected	
4.1.7 ▲	Select a model for evaluation	4.1.5 ▲	Select an evaluation design model and the types of data to be collected	
4.1.8 ▲	Develop data collection procedures for evaluation	4.1.6 ▲	Develop a sampling plan and procedures for data collection, management, and security	
4.1.9 ■	Develop data analysis plan for evaluation	4.1.6 ▲	Develop a sampling plan and procedures for data collection, management, and security	
4.1.10 ▲	Apply ethical principles to the evaluation process	8.1.1	Apply professional codes of ethics and ethical principles throughout assessment, planning, implementation, evaluation and research, communication, consulting, and advocacy processes	

Appendix B.1: Comparison of the Competencies and Sub-competencies of the HESPA I 2015 Model to the HESPA II 2020 Model

Key: Entry level = No symbol; Advanced-1 (▲); Advanced-2 (■)
Sub-competency worded the same in both Frameworks is indicated under comments

HESPA I Code	HESPA I 2015	HESPA II Code	HESPA II 2020	Comments
	Area IV: Conduct Evaluation and Research Related to Health Education/Promotion			
4.2	**Develop a research plan for health education/promotion**			
4.2.1 ■	Create statement of purpose	4.2.1 ■	Determine purpose, hypotheses, and questions	
4.2.2 ■	Assess feasibility of conducting research	4.2.4 ■	Assess capacity to conduct research	
4.2.3 ■	Conduct search for related literature	1.2.3	Conduct a literature review	
4.2.4 ■	Analyze and synthesize information found in the literature	1.2.3	Conduct a literature review	
4.2.5 ■	Develop research questions and/or hypotheses	4.2.1 ■	Determine purpose, hypotheses, and questions	
4.2.6 ■	Assess the merits and limitations of qualitative and quantitative data collection	4.2.7 ▲	Select quantitative and qualitative tools consistent with assumptions and data requirements	
4.2.7 ■	Select research design to address the research questions	4.2.5 ▲	Select a research design model and the types of data to be collected	
4.2.8 ■	Determine suitability of existing data collection instruments	4.2.7 ▲	Select quantitative and qualitative tools consistent with assumptions and data requirements	
4.2.9 ■	Identify research participants	4.2.6 ▲	Develop a sampling plan and procedures for data collection, management, and security	
4.2.10 ■	Develop sampling plan to select participants	4.2.6 ▲	Develop a sampling plan and procedures for data collection, management, and security	
4.2.11 ■	Develop data collection procedures for research	4.2.6 ▲	Develop a sampling plan and procedures for data collection, management, and security	
4.2.12 ■	Develop data analysis plan for research	4.2.6 ▲	Develop a sampling plan and procedures for data collection, management, and security	

APPENDIX B1

Appendix B.1: Comparison of the Competencies and Sub-competencies of the HESPA I 2015 Model to the HESPA II 2020 Model

Key: Entry level = No symbol; Advanced-1 (▲); Advanced-2 (■)
  Sub-competency worded the same in both Frameworks is indicated under comments

HESPA I Code	HESPA I 2015	HESPA II Code	HESPA II 2020	Comments
	Area IV: Conduct Evaluation and Research Related to Health Education/Promotion			
4.2.13 ■	Develop a plan for non-respondent follow-up	4.2.6 ▲	Develop a sampling plan and procedures for data collection, management, and security	
4.2.14 ■	Apply ethical principles to the research process	8.1.1	Apply professional codes of ethics and ethical principles throughout assessment, planning, implementation, evaluation and research, communication, consulting, and advocacy processes	
4.3	**Select, adapt and/or create instruments to collect data**			
4.3.1 ■	Identify existing data collection instruments	4.1.7 ▲ 4.2.7 ▲	Select quantitative and qualitative tools consistent with assumptions and data requirements Select quantitative and qualitative tools consistent with assumptions and data requirements	
4.3.2 ■	Adapt/modify existing data collection instruments	4.1.8 4.2.8 ■	Adopt, or modify instruments for collecting data Adopt, adapt, and/or develop instruments for collecting data	
4.3.3 ■	Create new data collection instruments	4.1.8 4.2.8 ■	Adopt, or modify instruments for collecting data Adopt, adapt, and/or develop instruments for collecting data	
4.3.4	Identify useable items from existing instruments	4.1.8 4.2.8 ■	Adopt, or modify instruments for collecting data Adopt, adapt, and/or develop instruments for collecting data	
4.3.5	Adapt/modify existing items	4.1.8 4.2.8 ■	Adopt, or modify instruments for collecting data Adopt, adapt, and/or develop instruments for collecting data	
4.3.6 ■	Create new items to be used in data collection	4.1.8 4.2.8 ■	Adopt, or modify instruments for collecting data Adopt, adapt, and/or develop instruments for collecting data	

Appendix B.1: Comparison of the Competencies and Sub-competencies of the HESPA I 2015 Model to the HESPA II 2020 Model

Key: Entry level = No symbol; Advanced-1 (▲); Advanced-2 (■)
Sub-competency worded the same in both Frameworks is indicated under comments

HESPA I Code	HESPA I 2015	HESPA II Code	HESPA II 2020	Comments
	Area IV: Conduct Evaluation and Research Related to Health Education/Promotion			
4.3.7 ■	Pilot test data collection instrument	4.2.9 ■	Implement a pilot test to refine and validate data collection instruments and procedures	
		4.1.10 ▲	Implement a pilot test to refine data collection instruments and procedures	
4.3.8 ■	Establish validity of data collection instruments	4.2.9 ■	Implement a pilot test to refine and validate data collection instruments and procedures	
4.3.9 ■	Ensure that data collection instruments generate reliable data	4.2.9 ■	Implement a pilot test to refine and validate data collection instruments and procedures	
4.3.10 ■	Ensure fairness of data collection instruments (for example, reduce bias, use language appropriate to priority population)	4.2.9 ■	Implement a pilot test to refine and validate data collection instruments and procedures	
		8.1.6	Apply principles of cultural humility, inclusion, and diversity in all aspects of practice (e.g., Culturally and Linguistically Appropriate Services (CLAS) standards and culturally responsive pedagogy)	
4.4	**Collect and manage data**			
4.4.1 ■	Train data collectors involved in evaluation and/or research	4.3.1 ■	Train data collectors	
4.4.2 ■	Collect data based on the evaluation or research plan	4.3.2	Implement data collection procedures	
4.4.3	Monitor and manage data collection	4.3.3	Use appropriate modalities to collect and manage data	
		4.3.4 ■	Monitor data collection procedures	
4.4.4	Use available technology to collect, monitor and manage data	4.3.3	Use appropriate modalities to collect and manage data	

Appendix B.1: Comparison of the Competencies and Sub-competencies of the HESPA I 2015 Model to the HESPA II 2020 Model

Key: Entry level = No symbol; Advanced-1 (▲); Advanced-2 (■)
   Sub-competency worded the same in both Frameworks is indicated under comments

HESPA I Code	HESPA I 2015	HESPA II Code	HESPA II 2020	Comments
	Area IV: Conduct Evaluation and Research Related to Health Education/Promotion			**Comments**
4.4.5	Comply with laws and regulations when collecting, storing, and protecting participant data	8.1.3 4.1.2 4.2.2 ▲	Comply with legal standards and regulatory guidelines in assessment, planning, implementation, evaluation and research, advocacy, management, communication, and reporting processes Comply with institutional requirements for evaluation Comply with institutional and/or IRB requirements for research	
4.5	**Analyze data**			
4.5.1 ■	Prepare data for analysis	4.3.5	Prepare data for analysis	Same wording
4.5.2 ▲	Analyze data using qualitative methods	4.3.6 ■	Analyze data	
4.5.3 ■	Analyze data using descriptive statistical methods	4.3.6 ■	Analyze data	
4.5.4 ■	Analyze data using inferential statistical methods	4.3.6 ■	Analyze data	
4.5.5 ■	Use technology to analyze data	4.3.6 ■	Analyze data	
4.6	**Interpret results**			
4.6.1 ■	Synthesize the analyzed data	4.4.6 ■	Synthesize findings	
4.6.2 ■	Explain how the results address the questions and/or hypotheses	4.4.1 ■	Explain how findings address the questions and/or hypotheses	
4.6.3 ■	Compare findings to results from other studies or evaluations	4.4.2 ▲	Compare findings to other evaluations or studies	
4.6.4 ■	Propose possible explanations of findings	4.4.4 ■	Draw conclusions based on findings	

Appendix B.1: Comparison of the Competencies and Sub-competencies of the HESPA I 2015 Model to the HESPA II 2020 Model

Key: Entry level = No symbol; Advanced-1 (▲); Advanced-2 (■)
Sub-competency worded the same in both Frameworks is indicated under comments

HESPA I Code	HESPA I 2015	HESPA II Code	HESPA II 2020	Comments
	Area IV: Conduct Evaluation and Research Related to Health Education/Promotion			
4.6.5 ■	Identify limitations of findings	4.4.3	Identify limitations and delimitations of findings	
4.6.6 ■	Address delimitations as they relate to findings	4.4.3	Identify limitations and delimitations of findings	
4.6.7 ■	Draw conclusions based on findings	4.4.4 ■	Draw conclusions based on findings	Same wording
4.6.8 ■	Develop recommendations based on findings	4.4.7 ■	Develop recommendations based on findings	Same wording
		4.5.3 ■	Identify recommendations for quality improvement	
		4.5.4 ▲	Translate findings into practice and interventions	
4.7	**Apply findings**			
4.7.1	Communicate findings to priority populations, partners, and stakeholders	4.5.1 ▲	Communicate findings by preparing reports and presentations, and by other means	
4.7.2	Solicit feedback from priority populations, partners, and stakeholders	1.1.5	Recruit and/or engage priority population(s), partners, and stakeholders to participate throughout all steps in the assessment, planning, implementation, and evaluation processes	
4.7.3	Evaluate feasibility of implementing recommendations	4.4.8 ■	Evaluate feasibility of implementing recommendations	Same wording
4.7.4	Incorporate findings into program improvement and refinement	4.5.3 ■	Identify recommendations for quality improvement	
		4.5.4 ▲	Translate findings into practice and interventions	
4.7.5 ■	Disseminate findings using a variety of methods	4.5.2 ■	Disseminate findings	

Appendix B.1: Comparison of the Competencies and Sub-competencies of the HESPA I 2015 Model to the HESPA II 2020 Model

Key: Entry level = No symbol; Advanced-1 (▲); Advanced-2 (■)

Sub-competency worded the same in both Frameworks is indicated under comments

HESPA I Code	HESPA I 2015	HESPA II Code	HESPA II 2020	
	Area V: Administer and Manage Health Education/Promotion			**Comments**
5.1	**Manage financial resources for health education/promotion programs**			
5.1.1 ▲	Develop financial plan	7.4.2 ▲	Develop financial budgets and plans	
5.1.2 ▲	Evaluate financial needs and resources	7.4.1 ▲	Evaluate internal and external financial needs and funding sources	
5.1.3 ▲	Identify internal and/or external funding sources	7.4.1 ▲	Evaluate internal and external financial needs and funding sources	
5.1.4 ▲	Prepare budget requests	7.4.2 ▲	Develop financial budgets and plans	
5.1.5 ▲	Develop program budgets	7.4.2 ▲	Develop financial budgets and plans	
5.1.6 ▲	Manage program budgets	7.4.3 ▲	Monitor budget performance	
5.1.7 ▲	Conduct cost analysis for programs	7.4.4 ■	Justify value of health education and promotion using economic (e.g., cost-benefit, return-on-investment, and value-on-investment) and/or other analyses	
5.1.8 ▲	Prepare budget reports			No match
5.1.9 ▲	Monitor financial plan	7.4.3 ▲	Monitor budget performance	
5.1.10 ▲	Create requests for funding proposals	7.4.5 ▲	Write grants and funding proposals	
5.1.11 ▲	Write grant proposals	7.4.5 ▲	Write grants and funding proposals	
5.1.12 ▲	Conduct reviews of funding proposals	7.4.6 ■	Conduct reviews of funding and grant proposals	
5.1.13 ▲	Apply ethical principles when managing financial resources	8.1.1	Apply professional codes of ethics and ethical principles throughout assessment, planning, implementation, evaluation and research, communication, consulting, and advocacy processes	

Appendix B.1: Comparison of the Competencies and Sub-competencies of the HESPA I 2015 Model to the HESPA II 2020 Model

Key: Entry level = No symbol; Advanced-1 (▲); Advanced-2 (■)
Sub-competency worded the same in both Frameworks is indicated under comments

HESPA I Code	HESPA I 2015	HESPA II Code	HESPA II 2020	Comments
	Area V: Administer and Manage Health Education/Promotion			Comments
5.2	**Manage technology resources**			
5.2.1	Assess technology needs to support health education/promotion			No match
5.2.2	Use technology to collect, store and retrieve program management data	7.4.8 ▲	Maintain up-to-date technology infrastructure	
5.2.3	Apply ethical principles in managing technology resources	8.1.1	Apply professional codes of ethics and ethical principles throughout assessment, planning, implementation, evaluation and research, communication, consulting, and advocacy processes	
5.2.4	Evaluate emerging technologies for applicability to health education/ promotion	7.4.8 ▲	Maintain up-to-date technology infrastructure	
5.3	**Manage relationships with partners and other stakeholders**			
5.3.1	Assess capacity of partners and other stakeholders to meet program goals	7.1.2	Assess the capacity of potential partners and stakeholders	
5.3.2 ▲	Facilitate discussions with partners and other stakeholders regarding program resource needs	7.1.3	Involve partners and stakeholders throughout the health education and promotion process in meaningful and sustainable ways	
5.3.3	Create agreements (for example, memoranda of understanding) with partners and other stakeholders	7.1.4 ▲	Execute formal and informal agreements with partners and stakeholders	
5.3.4	Monitor relationships with partners and other stakeholders	7.1.5	Evaluate relationships with partners and stakeholders on an ongoing basis to make appropriate modifications	
5.3.5 ▲	Elicit feedback from partners and other stakeholders	7.1.3 7.1.5	Involve partners and stakeholders throughout the health education and promotion process in meaningful and sustainable ways Evaluate relationships with partners and stakeholders on an ongoing basis to make appropriate modifications	

APPENDIX B1

Appendix B.1: Comparison of the Competencies and Sub-competencies of the HESPA I 2015 Model to the HESPA II 2020 Model

Key: Entry level = No symbol; Advanced-1 (▲); Advanced-2 (■)
Sub-competency worded the same in both Frameworks is indicated under comments

HESPA I Code	HESPA I 2015	HESPA II Code	HESPA II 2020	Comments
	Area V: Administer and Manage Health Education/Promotion			**Comments**
5.3.6	Evaluate relationships with partners and other stakeholders	7.1.5	Evaluate relationships with partners and stakeholders on an ongoing basis to make appropriate modifications	
5.4	**Gain acceptance and support for health education/promotion programs**			
5.4.1	Demonstrate how programs align with organizational structure, mission, and goals			No match
5.4.2	Identify evidence to justify programs	7.4.4 ■	Justify value of health education and promotion using economic (e.g., cost-benefit, return-on-investment, and value-on-investment) and/or other analyses	
5.4.3	Create a rationale to gain or maintain program support	7.4.4 ■ 2.1.3	Justify value of health education and promotion using economic (e.g., cost-benefit, return-on-investment, and value-on-investment) and/or other analyses Establish the rationale for the intervention	
5.4.4	Use various communication strategies to present rationale	6.3.2	Develop persuasive communications (e.g. storytelling, and program rationale)	
5.5	**Demonstrate leadership**			
5.5.1 ▲	Facilitate efforts to achieve organizational mission	7.5.1 ▲	Facilitate the development of strategic and/or improvement plans using systems thinking to promote the mission, vision, and goal statements for health education and promotion	
5.5.2	Analyze an organization's culture to determine the extent to which it supports health education/promotion	7.3.2 ▲	Facilitate positive organizational culture and climate	

Appendix B.1: Comparison of the Competencies and Sub-competencies of the HESPA I 2015 Model to the HESPA II 2020 Model

Key: Entry level = No symbol; Advanced-1 (▲); Advanced-2 (■)
Sub-competency worded the same in both Frameworks is indicated under comments.

HESPA I Code	HESPA I 2015	HESPA II Code	HESPA II 2020	Comments
	Area V: Administer and Manage Health Education/Promotion			
5.5.3	Develop strategies to reinforce or change organizational culture to support health education/promotion	7.3.2 ▲ 7.5.2 ▲	Facilitate positive organizational culture and climate Gain organizational acceptance for strategic and/or improvement plans	
5.5.4 ▲	Facilitate needed changes to organizational culture	7.3.2 ▲ 7.5.1 ▲	Facilitate positive organizational culture and climate Facilitate the development of strategic and/or improvement plans using systems thinking to promote the mission, vision, and goal statements for health education and promotion	
5.5.5 ▲	Conduct strategic planning	7.5.1 ▲	Facilitate the development of strategic and/or improvement plans using systems thinking to promote the mission, vision, and goal statements for health education and promotion	
5.5.6 ▲	Implement strategic plan	7.5.3 ▲	Implement the strategic plan, incorporating status updates and making refinements as appropriate	
5.5.7 ▲	Monitor strategic plan	7.5.3 ▲	Implement the strategic plan, incorporating status updates and making refinements as appropriate	
5.5.8	Conduct program quality assurance/ process improvement	3.3.4 7.5.3 ▲	Ensure plan is implemented with fidelity Implement the strategic plan, incorporating status updates and making refinements as appropriate	
5.5.9	Comply with existing laws and regulations	8.1.3	Comply with legal standards and regulatory guidelines in assessment, planning, implementation, evaluation and research, advocacy, management, communication, and reporting processes	

Appendix B.1: Comparison of the Competencies and Sub-competencies of the HESPA I 2015 Model to the HESPA II 2020 Model

Key: Entry level = No symbol; Advanced-1 (▲); Advanced-2 (■)
Sub-competency worded the same in both Frameworks is indicated under comments

HESPA I Code	HESPA I 2015	HESPA II Code	HESPA II 2020	Comments
	Area V: Administer and Manage Health Education/Promotion			**Comments**
5.5.10	Adhere to ethical principles of the profession	8.1.1	Apply professional codes of ethics and ethical principles throughout assessment, planning, implementation, evaluation and research, communication, consulting, and advocacy processes	
5.6	**Manage human resources for health education/promotion programs**			
5.6.1 ▲	Assess staffing needs	7.2.2	Recruit staff and volunteers involved in implementation	
5.6.2 ▲	Develop job descriptions	7.3.3 ▲	Develop job descriptions to meet staffing needs	
5.6.3 ▲	Apply human resource policies consistent with laws and regulations	8.1.3	Comply with legal standards and regulatory guidelines in assessment, planning, implementation, evaluation and research, advocacy, management, communication, and reporting processes	
5.6.4 ▲	Evaluate qualifications of staff members and volunteers needed for programs	7.3.3 ▲	Develop job descriptions to meet staffing needs	
5.6.5	Recruit staff members and volunteers for programs	1.1.5	Recruit and/or engage priority population(s), partners, and stakeholders to participate throughout all steps in the assessment, planning, implementation, and evaluation processes	
		7.3.4 ▲	Recruit qualified staff (including paraprofessionals) and volunteers	
		7.2.2	Recruit staff and volunteers involved in implementation	
5.6.6 ▲	Determine staff member and volunteer professional development needs	7.3.5 ▲	Evaluate performance of staff and volunteers formally and informally	
5.6.7 ▲	Develop strategies to enhance staff member and volunteer professional development	7.3.6 ▲	Provide professional development and training for staff and volunteers	

APPENDIX B1

Appendix B.1: Comparison of the Competencies and Sub-competencies of the HESPA I 2015 Model to the HESPA II 2020 Model

Key: Entry level = No symbol; Advanced-1 (▲); Advanced-2 (■)
Sub-competency worded the same in both Frameworks is indicated under comments

HESPA I Code	HESPA I 2015	HESPA II Code	HESPA II 2020	
	Area V: Administer and Manage Health Education/Promotion			**Comments**
5.6.8 ▲	Implement strategies to enhance the professional development of staff members and volunteers	7.3.6 ▲	Provide professional development and training for staff and volunteers	
5.6.9 ▲	Develop and implement strategies to retain staff members and volunteers	7.3.7 ▲ 7.3.8 ▲	Facilitate the engagement and retention of staff and volunteers Apply team building and conflict resolution techniques as appropriate	
5.6.10 ▲	Employ conflict resolution techniques	7.3.8 ▲	Apply team building and conflict resolution techniques as appropriate	
5.6.11 ▲	Facilitate team development	7.3.8 ▲	Apply team building and conflict resolution techniques as appropriate	
5.6.12 ▲	Evaluate performance of staff members and volunteers	7.3.5 ▲	Evaluate performance of staff and volunteers formally and informally	
5.6.13 ▲	Monitor performance and/or compliance of funding recipients	7.4.7 ▲	Monitor performance and/or compliance of funding recipients	Same wording
5.6.14 ▲	Apply ethical principles when managing human resources	8.1.1	Apply professional codes of ethics and ethical principles throughout assessment, planning, implementation, evaluation and research, communication, consulting, and advocacy processes	
	Area VI: Serve as a Health Education/Promotion Resource Person			**Comments**
6.1	**Obtain and disseminate health-related information**			
6.1.1	Assess needs for health-related information	6.1.2	Identify the assets, needs, and characteristics of the audience(s) that affect communication and message design (e.g., literacy levels, language, culture, and cognitive and perceptual abilities)	

Appendix B.1: Comparison of the Competencies and Sub-competencies of the HESPA I 2015 Model to the HESPA II 2020 Model

Key: Entry level = No symbol; Advanced-1 (▲); Advanced-2 (■)
Sub-competency worded the same in both Frameworks is indicated under comments

HESPA I Code	HESPA I 2015	HESPA II Code	HESPA II 2020	Comments
	Area VI: Serve as a Health Education/Promotion Resource Person			
6.1.2	Identify valid information resources	1.2.1 6.3.4	Identify primary data, secondary data, and evidence-informed resources Employ media literacy skills (e.g., identifying credible sources and balancing multiple viewpoints)	
6.1.3	Evaluate resource materials for accuracy, relevance, and timeliness	6.4.4	Assess the suitability of new and/or existing communication aids, materials, or tools for audience(s) (e.g., the CDC Clear Communication Index and the Suitability Assessment of Materials [SAM])	
6.1.4	Adapt information for consumer	6.3.3	Tailor message(s) for the audience(s)	
6.1.5	Convey health-related information to consumer	6.5.1 6.5.2 6.5.5	Deliver presentation(s) tailored to the audience(s) Use public speaking skills Deliver oral and written communication that aligns with professional standards of grammar, punctuation, and style	
6.2	**Train others to use health education/promotion skills**			
6.2.1 ▲	Assess training needs of potential participants	7.2.3 ▲	Assess training needs	
6.2.2 ▲	Develop a plan for conducting training	7.2.4 ▲	Plan training, including technical assistance and support	
6.2.3 ▲	Identify resources needed to conduct training	7.2.4 ▲	Plan training, including technical assistance and support	
6.2.4 ▲	Implement planned training	7.2.5 ▲	Implement training	
6.2.5 ▲	Conduct formative and summative evaluations of training	7.2.6 ▲	Evaluate training as appropriate throughout the process	
6.2.6 ▲	Use evaluative feedback to create future trainings	7.2.6 ▲	Evaluate training as appropriate throughout the process	

Appendix B.1: Comparison of the Competencies and Sub-competencies of the HESPA I 2015 Model to the HESPA II 2020 Model

Key: Entry level = No symbol; Advanced-1 (▲); Advanced-2 (■)
Sub-competency worded the same in both Frameworks is indicated under comments

HESPA I Code	HESPA I 2015	HESPA II Code	HESPA II 2020	Comments
	Area VI: Serve as a Health Education/Promotion Resource Person			**Comments**
6.3	**Provide advice and consultation on health education/promotion issues**			
6.3.1 ▲	Assess and prioritize requests for advice/ consultation	8.2.1 ▲	Evaluate personal and organizational capacity to provide consultation	
6.3.2 ▲	Establish advisory/consultative relationships	8.3.4	Build relationships with other professionals within and outside the profession	
6.3.3 ▲	Provide expert assistance and guidance	8.2.2 ▲	Provide expert consultation, assistance, and guidance to individuals, groups, and organizations	
6.3.4 ▲	Evaluate the effectiveness of the expert assistance provided	8.1.1	Apply professional codes of ethics and ethical principles throughout assessment, planning, implementation, evaluation and research, communication, consulting, and advocacy processes	
6.3.5 ▲	Apply ethical principles in consultative relationships	8.1.1	Apply professional codes of ethics and ethical principles throughout assessment, planning, implementation, evaluation and research, communication, consulting, and advocacy processes	
	Area VII: Communicate, Promote, and Advocate for Health, Health Education/Promotion, and the Profession			**Comments**
7.1	**Identify, develop, and deliver messages using a variety of communication strategies, methods, and techniques**			
7.1.1	Create messages using communication theories and/or models	8.1.5 6.3.1	Use evidence-informed theories, models, and strategies Use communications theory to develop or select communication message(s)	

APPENDIX B1

Appendix B.1: Comparison of the Competencies and Sub-competencies of the HESPA I 2015 Model to the HESPA II 2020 Model

Key: Entry level = No symbol; Advanced-1 (▲); Advanced-2 (■)
Sub-competency worded the same in both Frameworks is indicated under comments

HESPA I Code	HESPA I 2015	HESPA II Code	HESPA II 2020	Comments
	Area VII: Communicate, Promote, and Advocate for Health, Health Education/Promotion, and the Profession			Comments
7.1.2	Identify level of literacy of intended audience	1.3.2	Determine the knowledge, attitudes, beliefs, skills, and behaviors that impact the health and health literacy of the priority population(s)	
		6.1.2	Identify the assets, needs, and characteristics of the audience(s) that affect communication and message design (e.g., literacy levels, language, culture, and cognitive and perceptual abilities)	
7.1.3	Tailor messages for intended audience	6.3.3	Tailor message(s) for the audience(s)	Same wording
7.1.4 ▲	Pilot test messages and delivery methods	6.4.5	Pilot test message(s) and communication aids, materials, or tools	
7.1.5 ▲	Revise messages based on pilot feedback	6.4.6	Revise communication aids, materials, or tools based on pilot results	
7.1.6	Assess and select methods and technologies used to deliver messages	6.1.3	Identify communication channels (e.g., social media and mass media) available to and used by the audience(s)	
		6.4.1	Differentiate the strengths and weaknesses of various communication channels and technologies (e.g., mass media, community mobilization, counseling, peer communication, information/digital technology, and apps)	
		6.4.2	Select communication channels and current and emerging technologies that are most appropriate for the audience(s) and message(s)	
		6.4.3	Develop communication aids, materials, or tools using appropriate multimedia (e.g., infographics, presentation software, brochures, and posters)	

Appendix B.1: Comparison of the Competencies and Sub-competencies of the HESPA I 2015 Model to the HESPA II 2020 Model

Key: Entry level = No symbol; Advanced-1 (▲); Advanced-2 (■)
Sub-competency worded the same in both Frameworks is indicated under comments

HESPA I Code	HESPA I 2015	HESPA II Code	HESPA II 2020	Comments
	Area VII: Communicate, Promote, and Advocate for Health, Health Education/Promotion, and the Profession			
7.1.7	Deliver messages using media and communication strategies	6.5.1	Deliver presentation(s) tailored to the audience(s)	
		6.5.4	Use current and emerging communication tools and trends (e.g., social media)	
		6.5.5	Deliver oral and written communication that aligns with professional standards of grammar, punctuation, and style	
		6.5.6	Use digital media to engage audience(s) (e.g., social media management tools and platforms)	
7.1.8	Evaluate the impact of the delivered messages	6.6.1	Conduct process, and impact evaluations of communications	
		6.6.2 ■	Conduct outcome evaluations of communications	
		6.6.3 ▲	Assess reach and dose of communication using tools (e.g., data mining software, social media analytics, and website analytics)	
7.2	**Engage in advocacy for health and health education/promotion**			
7.2.1	Identify current and emerging issues requiring advocacy	5.1.1	Examine the determinants of health and their underlying causes (e.g., poverty, trauma, and population-based discrimination) related to identified health issues	
		5.1.2	Examine evidence-informed findings related to identified health issues and desired changes	
7.2.2	Engage stakeholders in advocacy initiatives	5.2.3 ▲	Create formal and/or informal alliances, task forces, and coalitions to address the proposed change	
		5.2.4	Educate stakeholders on the health issue and the proposed policy, system, or environmental change	
		5.1.5	Identify existing coalition(s) or stakeholders that can be engaged in advocacy efforts	

Appendix B.1: Comparison of the Competencies and Sub-competencies of the HESPA I 2015 Model to the HESPA II 2020 Model

Key: Entry level = No symbol; Advanced-1 (▲); Advanced-2 (■)

Sub-competency worded the same in both Frameworks is indicated under comments

HESPA I Code	HESPA I 2015	HESPA II Code	HESPA II 2020	Comments
	Area VII: Communicate, Promote, and Advocate for Health, Health Education/Promotion, and the Profession			
7.2.3	Access resources (for example, financial, personnel, information, data) related to identified advocacy needs	5.2.5	Identify available resources and gaps (e.g., financial, personnel, information, and data)	
7.2.4	Develop advocacy plans in compliance with local, state, and/or federal policies and procedures	5.2.6	Identify organizational policies and procedures and federal, state, and local laws that pertain to the advocacy efforts	
		5.2.8	Specify strategies, a timeline, and roles and responsibilities to address the proposed policy, system, or environmental change (e.g., develop ongoing relationships with decision makers and stakeholders, use social media, register others to vote, and seek political appointment)	
		8.1.3	Comply with legal standards and regulatory guidelines in assessment, planning, implementation, evaluation and research, advocacy, management, communication, and reporting processes	
7.2.5	Use strategies that advance advocacy goals	5.2.7	Develop persuasive messages and materials (e.g., briefs, resolutions, and fact sheets) to communicate the policy, system, or environmental change	
		5.2.8	Specify strategies, a timeline, and roles and responsibilities to address the proposed policy, system, or environmental change (e.g., develop ongoing relationships with decision makers and stakeholders, use social media, register others to vote, and seek political appointment)	
		5.3.1	Use media to conduct advocacy (e.g., social media, press releases, public service announcements, and op-eds)	
		5.3.2	Use traditional, social, and emerging technologies and methods to mobilize support for policy, system, or environmental change	
		5.3.3 ▲	Sustain coalitions and stakeholder relationships to achieve and maintain policy, system, or environmental change	

Appendix B.1: Comparison of the Competencies and Sub-competencies of the HESPA I 2015 Model to the HESPA II 2020 Model

Key: Entry level = No symbol; Advanced-1 (▲); Advanced-2 (■)
 Sub-competency worded the same in both Frameworks is indicated under comments

HESPA I Code	HESPA I 2015	HESPA II Code	HESPA II 2020	Comments
	Area VII: Communicate, Promote, and Advocate for Health, Health Education/Promotion, and the Profession			
7.2.6	Implement advocacy plans	5.3.1	Use media to conduct advocacy (e.g., social media, press releases, public service announcements, and op-eds)	
		5.3.2	Use traditional, social, and emerging technologies and methods to mobilize support for policy, system, or environmental change	
		5.3.3 ▲	Sustain coalitions and stakeholder relationships to achieve and maintain policy, system, or environmental change	
7.2.7	Evaluate advocacy efforts	5.4.1	Conduct process, impact, and outcome evaluation of advocacy efforts	
		5.4.2	Use the results of the evaluation to inform next steps	
7.2.8	Comply with organizational policies related to participating in advocacy	8.1.3	Comply with legal standards and regulatory guidelines in assessment, planning, implementation, evaluation and research, advocacy, management, communication, and reporting processes	
7.2.9	Lead advocacy initiatives related to health (Continued on p. 133)	5.2.8	Specify strategies, a timeline, and roles and responsibilities to address the proposed policy, system, or environmental change (e.g., develop ongoing relationships with decision makers and stakeholders, use social media, register others to vote, and seek political appointment)	
		5.2.3 ▲	Create formal and/or informal alliances, task forces, and coalitions to address the proposed change	
		5.3.3 ▲	Sustain coalitions and stakeholder relationships to achieve and maintain policy, system, or environmental change	

Appendix B.1: Comparison of the Competencies and Sub-competencies of the HESPA I 2015 Model to the HESPA II 2020 Model

Key: Entry level = No symbol; Advanced-1 (▲); Advanced-2 (■)
Sub-competency worded the same in both Frameworks is indicated under comments

HESPA I Code	HESPA I 2015	HESPA II Code	HESPA II 2020	Comments
	Area VII: Communicate, Promote, and Advocate for Health, Health Education/Promotion, and the Profession			
7.2.9	(Continued from p. 132) Lead advocacy initiatives related to health	7.1.3	Involve partners and stakeholders throughout the health education and promotion process in meaningful and sustainable ways	
		7.4.4 ■	Justify value of health education and promotion using economic (e.g., cost-benefit, return-on-investment, and value-on-investment) and/or other analyses	
7.3	**Influence policy and/or systems change to promote health and health education**			
7.3.1	Assess the impact of existing and proposed policies on health	5.1.1	Examine the determinants of health and their underlying causes (e.g., poverty, trauma, and population-based discrimination) related to identified health issues	
		5.2.6	Identify organizational policies and procedures and federal, state, and local laws that pertain to the advocacy efforts	
		1.3.4	Assess existing and available resources, policies, programs, practices, and interventions	
		1.3.3	Identify the social, cultural, economic, political, and environmental factors that impact the health and/or learning processes of the priority population(s)	
7.3.2	Assess the impact of existing and proposed policies on health education	5.2.6	Identify organizational policies and procedures and federal, state, and local laws that pertain to the advocacy efforts	
		1.3.4	Assess existing and available resources, policies, programs, practices, and interventions	

APPENDIX B1

Appendix B.1: Comparison of the Competencies and Sub-competencies of the HESPA I 2015 Model to the HESPA II 2020 Model

Key: Entry level = No symbol; Advanced-1 (▲); Advanced-2 (■)
   Sub-competency worded the same in both Frameworks is indicated under comments

HESPA I Code	HESPA I 2015	HESPA II Code	HESPA II 2020	Comments
	Area VII: Communicate, Promote, and Advocate for Health, Health Education/Promotion, and the Profession			Comments
7.3.3	Assess the impact of existing systems on health	5.1.1	Examine the determinants of health and their underlying causes (e.g., poverty, trauma, and population-based discrimination) related to identified health issues	
		1.3.3	Identify the social, cultural, economic, political, and environmental factors that impact the health and/or learning processes of the priority population(s)	
7.3.4	Project the impact of proposed systems changes on health education			No match
7.3.5	Use evidence-based findings in policy analysis	5.1.2	Examine evidence-informed findings related to identified health issues and desired changes	
7.3.6 ▲	Develop policies to promote health using evidence-based findings	8.1.5	Use evidence-informed theories, models and strategies	
7.3.7 ▲	Identify factors that influence decision-makers	5.2.2	Identify factors that influence decision-makers (e.g., societal and cultural norms, financial considerations, upcoming elections, and voting record)	
7.3.8 ▲	Use policy advocacy techniques to influence decision-makers (Continued on p. 135)	5.2.4	Educate stakeholders on the health issue and the proposed policy, system, or environmental change	
		5.2.7	Develop persuasive messages and materials (e.g., briefs, resolutions, and fact sheets) to communicate the policy, system, or environmental change	
		5.3.1	Use media to conduct advocacy (e.g., social media, press releases, public service announcements, and op-eds)	
		5.3.2	Use traditional, social, and emerging technologies and methods to mobilize support for policy, system, or environmental change	

APPENDIX B1

Appendix B.1: Comparison of the Competencies and Sub-competencies of the HESPA I 2015 Model to the HESPA II 2020 Model

Key: Entry level = No symbol; Advanced-1 (▲); Advanced-2 (■)
Sub-competency worded the same in both Frameworks is indicated under comments

HESPA I Code	HESPA I 2015	HESPA II Code	HESPA II 2020	Comments
	Area VII: Communicate, Promote, and Advocate for Health, Health Education/Promotion, and the Profession			
7.3.8 ▲	(Continued from p. 134) Use policy advocacy techniques to influence decision-makers	5.3.3 ▲ 6.5.1	Sustain coalitions and stakeholder relationships to achieve and maintain policy, system, or environmental change Deliver presentation(s) tailored to the audience(s)	
7.3.9	Use media advocacy techniques to influence decision-makers	5.3.1	Use media to conduct advocacy (e.g., social media, press releases, public service announcements, and op-eds)	
7.3.10	Engage in legislative advocacy	5.2.8 5.3.1 5.3.2	Specify strategies, a timeline, and roles and responsibilities to address the proposed policy, system, or environmental change (e.g., develop ongoing relationships with decision makers and stakeholders, use social media, register others to vote, and seek political appointment) Use media to conduct advocacy (e.g., social media, press releases, public service announcements, and op-eds) Use traditional, social, and emerging technologies and methods to mobilize support for policy, system, or environmental change	
7.4	**Promote the health education profession**			
7.4.1	Explain the major responsibilities of the health education specialist	8.4.1	Explain the major responsibilities, contributions, and value of the health education specialist	
7.4.2	Explain the role of professional organizations in advancing the profession	8.4.2	Explain the role of professional organizations and the benefits of participating in them	
7.4.3	Explain the benefits of participating in professional organizations	8.4.2	Explain the role of professional organizations and the benefits of participating in them	

Appendix B.1: Comparison of the Competencies and Sub-competencies of the HESPA I 2015 Model to the HESPA II 2020 Model

Key: Entry level = No symbol; Advanced-1 (▲); Advanced-2 (■)
 Sub-competency worded the same in both Frameworks is indicated under comments

HESPA I Code	HESPA I 2015	HESPA II Code	HESPA II 2020	Comments
	Area VII: Communicate, Promote, and Advocate for Health, Health Education/Promotion, and the Profession			Comments
7.4.4	Advocate for professional development of health education specialists	8.4.3	Advocate for professional development for health education specialists	Same wording
7.4.5	Advocate for the profession	8.4.3 / 8.4.4	Advocate for professional development for health education specialists / Educate others about the history of the profession, its current status, and its implications for professional practice	
7.4.6	Explain the history of the profession and its current and future implications for professional practice	8.4.4	Educate others about the history of the profession, its current status, and its implications for professional practice	
7.4.7	Explain the role of credentialing (for example, individual, program) in the promotion of the profession	8.4.5	Explain the role and benefits of credentialing (e.g., individual and program)	
7.4.8	Develop and implement a professional development plan	8.3.2 / 8.3.3	Participate in continuing education opportunities to maintain or enhance continuing competence / Develop a career advancement plan	
7.4.9 ■	Serve as a mentor to others in the profession	8.3.5 ■	Serve as a mentor	
7.4.10 ■	Develop materials that contribute to the professional literature	8.4.6 ▲	Develop presentations and publications that contribute to the professional literature	
7.4.11 ■	Engage in service to advance the profession	8.2.3 ■ / 8.3.1 / 8.4.7 ▲	Conduct peer reviews (e.g. manuscripts, abstracts, proposals, and tenure folios) / Participate in professional associations, coalitions, and networks (e.g. serving on committees, attending conferences, and providing leadership / Engage in service to advance the profession	Same wording

APPENDIX B1

Appendix B.2: Comparison of the Competencies and Sub-competencies of the HESPA II 2020 Model to the HESPA I 2015 Model

Table: B.2
Comparison of the HESPA II 2020 Model (New) to the HESPA I 2015 Model (Old)

Many of the HESPA I 2015 Sub-competencies correlate to similar HESPA II 2020 Sub-competencies. If the Sub-competency is worded the same in both Frameworks, it is indicated under comments. All advanced-1 Sub-competencies are indicated by the symbol (▲), and the advanced-2 Sub-competencies are indicated by the symbol (■). "No match" indicated no direct/similar Sub-competency.

Key: Entry level = No symbol; Advanced-1 (▲); Advanced-2 (■)
Sub-competency worded the same in both Frameworks is indicated under comments

HESPA II Code	HESPA II 2020	HESPA I Code	HESPA I 2015	Comments
	Area I: Assessment of Needs and Capacity			
1.1	**Plan assessment**	**1.1**	**Plan assessment process for health education/promotion**	
1.1.1	Define the purpose and scope of the assessment			No match
1.1.2	Identify priority population(s)	1.1.1 2.1.1	Define the priority population to be assessed Identify priority populations, partners, and other stakeholders	
1.1.3	Identify existing and available resources, policies, programs, practices, and interventions	1.1.2	Identify existing and necessary resources to conduct assessments	
1.1.4	Examine the factors and determinants that influence the assessment process	1.6.4	Assess social, environmental, political, and other factors that may impact health education/promotion	
1.1.5	Recruit and/or engage priority population(s), partners, and stakeholders to participate throughout all steps in the assessment, planning, implementation, and evaluation processes	1.1.3 3.2.2 4.7.2 5.6.5	Engage priority populations, partners, and stakeholders to participate in the assessment process Recruit individuals needed for implementation Solicit feedback from priority populations, partners, and stakeholders Recruit staff members and volunteers for programs	

Appendix B.2: Comparison of the Competencies and Sub-competencies of the HESPA II 2020 Model to the HESPA I 2015 Model

Key: Entry level = No symbol; Advanced-1 (▲); Advanced-2 (■)

Sub-competency worded the same in both Frameworks is indicated under comments

HESPA II Code	HESPA II 2020	HESPA I Code	HESPA I 2015	Comments
	Area I: Assessment of Needs and Capacity			**Comments**
1.2	**Obtain primary data, secondary data, and other evidence-informed sources**	**1.2** **1.3**	**Access existing information and data related to health** **Collect primary data to determine needs**	
1.2.1	Identify primary data, secondary data, and evidence-informed resources	1.2.1	Identify sources of secondary data related to health	
1.2.2 ▲	Establish collaborative relationships and agreements that facilitate access to data	1.2.2	Establish collaborative relationships and agreements that facilitate access to data	Same Wording
1.2.3	Conduct a literature review	1.2.3 4.2.3 ■ 4.2.4 ■	Review related literature Conduct search for related literature Analyze and synthesize information found in the literature	
1.2.4	Procure secondary data	1.2.5	Extract data from existing databases	
1.2.5	Determine the validity and reliability of the secondary data	1.2.6	Determine the validity of existing data	
1.2.6	Identify data gaps	1.2.4	Identify gaps in secondary data	
1.2.7	Determine primary data collection needs, instruments, methods, and procedures	1.3.1 1.3.2 1.3.3	Identify data collection instruments Select data collection methods for use in assessment Develop data collection procedures	
1.2.8	Adhere to established procedures to collect data	1.3.5	Implement quantitative and/or qualitative data collection	
1.2.9 ▲	Develop a data analysis plan			No match
1.3	**Analyze the data to determine the health of the priority population(s) and the factors that influence health**	**1.4** **1.5**	**Analyze relationships among behavioral, environmental, and other factors that influence health** **Examine factors that influence the process by which people learn**	
1.3.1	Determine the health status of the priority population(s)			No match

Appendix B.2: Comparison of the Competencies and Sub-competencies of the HESPA II 2020 Model to the HESPA I 2015 Model

Key: Entry level = No symbol; Advanced-1 (▲); Advanced-2 (■)
Sub-competency worded the same in both Frameworks is indicated under comments

HESPA II Code	HESPA II 2020	HESPA I Code	HESPA I 2015	Comments
	Area I: Assessment of Needs and Capacity			Comments
1.3.2	Determine the knowledge, attitudes, beliefs, skills, and behaviors that impact the health and health literacy of the priority population(s)	1.4.1	Identify and analyze factors that influence health behaviors	
		1.4.2	Identify and analyze factors that influence health	
		1.5.2	Identify and analyze factors that foster or hinder knowledge acquisition	
		1.5.3	Identify and analyze factors that influence attitudes and beliefs	
		1.5.4	Identify and analyze factors that foster or hinder acquisition of skills	
1.3.3	Identify the social, cultural, economic, political, and environmental factors that impact the health and/or learning processes of the priority population(s)	1.4.1	Identify and analyze factors that influence health behaviors	
		1.4.2	Identify and analyze factors that influence health	
		1.4.3	Identify the impact of emerging social, economic, and other trends on health	
		1.5.1	Identify and analyze factors that foster or hinder the learning process	
		1.5.2	Identify and analyze factors that foster or hinder knowledge acquisition	
		1.6.4	Assess social, environmental, political, and other factors that may impact health education/promotion	
		2.3.6	Identify delivery methods and settings to facilitate learning	
		7.3.3	Assess the impact of existing systems on health	
1.3.4	Assess existing and available resources, policies, programs, practices, and interventions	1.6.1	Determine the extent of available health education/promotion programs and interventions	
		1.6.2	Identify policies related to health education/promotion	
		1.6.3	Assess the effectiveness of existing health education/promotion programs and interventions	
		1.6.4	Assess social, environmental, political, and other factors that may impact health education/promotion	
		7.3.1	Assess the impact of existing and pro-posed policies on health	
		7.3.2	Assess the impact of existing and proposed policies on health education	

Appendix B.2: Comparison of the Competencies and Sub-competencies of the HESPA II 2020 Model to the HESPA I 2015 Model

Key: Entry level = No symbol; Advanced-1 (▲); Advanced-2 (■)
   Sub-competency worded the same in both Frameworks is indicated under comments

HESPA II Code	HESPA II 2020	HEPSA I Code	HESPA I 2015	Comments
	Area I: Assessment of Needs and Capacity			Comments
1.3.5	Determine the capacity (available resources, policies, programs, practices, and interventions) to improve and/or maintain health	1.6.1	Determine the extent of available health education/promotion programs and interventions	
		1.6.2	Identify policies related to health education/promotion	
		1.6.5	Analyze the capacity for providing necessary health education/promotion	
		1.7.2	Identify current needs, resources, and capacity	
1.3.6	List the needs of the priority population(s)	1.7.1	Synthesize assessment findings	
		1.7.2	Identify current needs, resources, and capacity	
1.4	**Synthesize assessment findings to inform the planning process**	**1.6**	**Examine factors that enhance or impede the process of health education/promotion**	
		1.7	**Determine needs for health education/promotion based on assessment findings**	
1.4.1 ▲	Compare findings to norms, existing data, and other information	1.7.1	Synthesize assessment findings	
1.4.2	Prioritize health education and promotion needs	1.7.3	Prioritize health education/promotion needs	Same wording
1.4.3	Summarize the capacity of priority population(s) to meet the needs of the priority population(s)			No match
1.4.4	Develop recommendations based on findings	1.7.4	Develop recommendations for health education/promotion based on assessment findings	
1.4.5	Report assessment findings	1.7.5	Report assessment findings	Same wording

Appendix B.2: Comparison of the Competencies and Sub-competencies of the HESPA II 2020 Model to the HESPA I 2015 Model

Key: Entry level = No symbol; Advanced-1 (▲); Advanced-2 (■)
Sub-competency worded the same in both Frameworks is indicated under comments

HESPA II Code	HESPA II 2020		HESPA I 2015		
	Area II: Planning				**Comments**
2.1	**Engage priority populations, partners, and stakeholders for participation in the planning process**	**2.1**	**Involve priority populations, partners, and other stakeholders in the planning process**		
2.1.1	Convene priority populations, partners, and stakeholders	2.1.1 2.1.2	Identify priority populations, partners and other stakeholders. Use strategies to convene priority populations, partners, and other stakeholders		
2.1.2	Facilitate collaborative efforts among priority populations, partners, and stakeholders	2.1.3	Facilitate collaborative efforts among priority populations, partners, and other stakeholders	Same wording	
2.1.3	Establish the rationale for the intervention	5.4.3	Create a rationale to gain or maintain program support		
2.2	**Define desired outcomes**	**2.2**	**Develop goals and objectives**		
2.2.1	Identify desired outcomes using the needs and capacity assessment	2.2.1	Identify desired outcomes using the needs assessment results		
2.2.2	Elicit input from priority populations, partners, and stakeholders regarding desired outcomes	2.1.4	Elicit input about the plan		
2.2.3	Develop vision, mission, and goal statements for the intervention(s)	2.2.2 2.2.3 2.2.4	Develop vision statement Develop mission statement Develop goal statements		
2.2.4	Develop specific, measurable, achievable, realistic, and time-bound (SMART) objectives)	2.2.5 3.2.1 ▲	Develop specific, measurable, attainable, realistic, and time-sensitive objectives Develop training objectives		
2.3	**Determine health education and promotion interventions**	**2.3**	**Select or design strategies/ interventions**		
2.3.1	Select planning model(s) for health education and promotion	2.3.1	Select planning model(s) for health education/promotion	Same Wording	
2.3.2 ▲	Create a logic model	2.4.1 2.4.3	Use theories and/or models to guide the delivery plan Organize health education/promotion into a logical sequence		

Appendix B.2: Comparison of the Competencies and Sub-competencies of the HESPA II 2020 Model to the HESPA I 2015 Model

Key: Entry level = No symbol; Advanced-1 (▲); Advanced-2 (■)
Sub-competency worded the same in both Frameworks is indicated under comments

HESPA II Code	HESPA II 2020	HESPA I Code	HESPA I 2015		Comments
	Area II: Planning				**Comments**
2.3.3 ▲	Assess the effectiveness and alignment of existing interventions to desired outcomes	2.3.2	Assess efficacy of various strategies/interventions to ensure consistency with objectives		
2.3.4	Adopt, adapt, and/or develop tailored intervention(s) for priority population(s) to achieve desired outcomes	2.3.7 / 2.3.8	Tailor strategies/interventions for priority populations / Adapt existing strategies/interventions as needed		
2.3.5 ▲	Plan for acquisition of required tools and resources	2.4.2 / 3.1.4	Identify the resources involved in the delivery of health education/promotion / Arrange for needed services to implement plan		
2.3.6 ▲	Conduct a pilot test of intervention(s)	2.3.9 / 2.4.10	Conduct pilot test of strategies/interventions / Design and conduct pilot study of health education/promotion plan		
2.3.7 ▲	Revise intervention(s) based on pilot feedback	2.3.10	Refine strategies/interventions based on pilot feedback		
2.4	**Develop plans and materials for implementation and evaluation**	**2.4** / **2.5**	**Develop a plan for the delivery of health education/promotion** / **Address factors that influence implementation of health education/ promotion**		
2.4.1 ▲	Develop an implementation plan inclusive of logic model, work plan, responsible parties, timeline, marketing, and communication	2.4.3 / 2.4.4	Organize health education/promotion into a logical sequence. / Develop a timeline for the delivery of health education/promotion		
2.4.2	Develop materials needed for implementation	2.4.5 / 3.1.2	Develop marketing plan to deliver health program / Develop materials to implement plan		
2.4.3	Address factors that influence implementation	2.5.1 / 2.5.2	Identify and analyze factors that foster or hinder implementation / Develop plans and processes to overcome potential barriers to implementation		
2.4.4 ▲	Plan for evaluation and dissemination of results				No match

Appendix B.2: Comparison of the Competencies and Sub-competencies of the HESPA II 2020 Model to the HESPA I 2015 Model

Key: Entry level = No symbol; Advanced-1 (▲); Advanced-2 (■)
Sub-competency worded the same in both Frameworks is indicated under comments

HESPA II Code	HESPA II 2020	HESPA I Code	HESPA I 2015	Comments
	Area II: Planning			**Comments**
2.4.5 ▲	Plan for sustainability	2.4.7	Analyze the opportunity for integrating health education/promotion into other programs	
		2.4.8	Develop a process for integrating health education/promotion into other pro-grams when needed	
		2.4.9	Assess the sustainability of the delivery plan	
	Area III: Implementation			
3.1	**Coordinate the delivery of intervention(s) consistent with the implementation plan**	**3.1**	**Coordinate the logistics necessary to implement plan**	
		3.2	**Train staff members and volunteers involved in implementation of health education/promotion**	
3.1.1	Secure implementation resources	3.1.3	Secure resources to implement plan	
3.1.2	Arrange for implementation services	3.1.4	Arrange for needed services to imple-ment plan	
3.1.3	Comply with contractual obligations	3.1.6	Comply with legal standards that apply to implementation	
3.1.4 ▲	Establish training protocol	3.2.1 ▲	Develop training objectives	
		3.2.3	Identify training needs of individuals involved in implementation	
		3.2.4	Develop training using best practices	
3.1.5	Train staff and volunteers to ensure fidelity	3.2.5	Implement training	
3.2	**Deliver health education and promotion interventions**	**3.3**	**Implement health education/ promotion plan**	
3.2.1	Create an environment conducive to learning	3.1.1	Create an environment conducive to learning	Same wording
3.2.2	Collect baseline data	3.3.1	Collect baseline data	Same wording
3.2.3	Implement a marketing plan	3.3.5	Implement marketing plan	Same wording
3.2.4	Deliver health education and promotion as designed	3.3.6	Deliver health education/promotion as designed	Same wording
3.2.5	Employ an appropriate variety of instructional methodologies	3.3.7	Use a variety of strategies to deliver plan	

Appendix B.2: Comparison of the Competencies and Sub-competencies of the HESPA II 2020 Model to the HESPA I 2015 Model

Key: Entry level = No symbol; Advanced-1 (▲); Advanced-2 (■)

Sub-competency worded the same in both Frameworks is indicated under comments

HESPA II Code	HESPA II 2020	HESPA I Code	HESPA I 2015	
	Area III: Implementation			**Comments**
3.3	**Monitor implementation**	**3.4**	**Monitor implementation of health education/promotion**	
3.3.1	Monitor progress in accordance with the timeline	3.4.1	Monitor progress in accordance with timeline	Same Wording
3.3.2	Assess progress in achieving objectives	3.4.2	Assess progress in achieving objectives	Same Wording
3.3.3	Modify interventions as needed to meet individual needs	3.4.4	Modify plan when needed	
3.3.4	Ensure plan is implemented with fidelity	3.4.3	Ensure plan is implemented consistently	
3.3.5	Monitor use of resources	3.4.5	Monitor use of resources	Same wording
3.3.6	Evaluate the sustainability of implementation	3.4.6	Evaluate sustainability of implementation	Same wording
	Area IV: Evaluation and Research			**Comments**
4.1	**Design process, impact, and outcome evaluation of the intervention**	**4.1** **4.3**	**Develop evaluation plan for health education/promotion** **Select/adapt and/or create instruments to collect data**	
4.1.1 ▲	Align the evaluation plan with the intervention goals and objectives	4.1.1	Determine the purpose and goals of evaluation	
4.1.2	Comply with institutional requirements for evaluation	4.4.5	Comply with laws and regulations when collecting, storing, and protecting participant data	
4.1.3 ▲	Use a logic model and/or theory for evaluations	4.1.3 4.1.4	Create a logic model to guide the evaluation process Adapt/modify a logic model to guide the evaluation process	
4.1.4 ▲	Assess capacity to conduct evaluation	4.1.5	Assess needed and available resources to conduct evaluation	

Appendix B.2: Comparison of the Competencies and Sub-competencies of the HESPA II 2020 Model to the HESPA I 2015 Model

Key: Entry level = No symbol; Advanced-1 (▲); Advanced-2 (■)
Sub-competency worded the same in both Frameworks is indicated under comments

HESPA II Code	HESPA II 2020	HESPA I Code	HESPA I 2015	
	Area IV: Evaluation and Research			**Comments**
4.1.5 ▲	Select an evaluation design model and the types of data to be collected	4.1.2 4.1.6 4.1.7	Develop questions to be answered by the evaluation Determine the types of data (for example, qualitative, quantitative) to be collected Select a model for evaluation	
4.1.6 ▲	Develop a sampling plan and procedures for data collection, management, and security	4.1.8 4.1.9 ■	Develop data collection procedures for evaluation Develop data analysis plan for evaluation	
4.1.7 ▲	Select quantitative and qualitative tools consistent with assumptions and data requirements	4.3.1	Identify existing data collection instruments	
4.1.8	Adopt or modify existing instruments for collecting data	4.3.2 4.3.4 4.3.5	Adapt/modify existing data collection instruments Identify useable items from existing instruments Adapt/modify existing items	
4.1.9 ▲	Develop instruments for collecting data	4.3.3 ■ 4.3.6 ■	Create new data collection instruments Create new items to be used in data collection	
4.1.10 ▲	Implement a pilot test to refine data collection instruments and procedures	4.3.7 ■	Pilot test data collection instrument	
4.2	**Design research studies**	**4.2**	**Develop a research plan for health education/promotion**	
4.2.1 ■	Determine purpose, hypotheses, and questions	4.2.1 4.2.5	Create statement of purpose Develop research questions and/or hypotheses	
4.2.2 ▲	Comply with institutional and/or IRB requirements for research	4.4.5 4.2.14	Comply with laws and regulations when collecting, storing, and protecting participant data Apply ethical principles to the research process	

Appendix B.2: Comparison of the Competencies and Sub-competencies of the HESPA II 2020 Model to the HESPA I 2015 Model

Key: Entry level = No symbol; Advanced-1 (▲); Advanced-2 (■)

    Sub-competency worded the same in both Frameworks is indicated under comments

HESPA II Code	HESPA II 2020	HESPA I Code	HESPA I 2015		Comments
	Area IV: Evaluation and Research				**Comments**
4.2.3 ▲	Use a logic model and/or theory for research				No match
4.2.4 ■	Assess capacity to conduct research	4.2.2	Assess feasibility of conducting research		
4.2.5 ▲	Select a research design model and the types of data to be collected	4.2.7	Select research design to address the research questions		
4.2.6 ▲	Develop a sampling plan and procedures for data collection, management, and security	4.2.9 4.2.10 4.2.11 4.2.12 ■ 4.2.13	Identify research participants Develop sampling plan to select participants Develop data collection procedures for research Develop data analysis plan for research Develop a plan for non-respondent follow-up		
4.2.7 ▲	Select quantitative and qualitative tools consistent with assumptions and data requirements	4.2.6 4.2.8 4.3.1	Assess the merits and limitations of qualitative and quantitative data collection Determine suitability of existing data collection instruments Identify existing data collection instruments		
4.2.8 ■	Adopt, adapt, and/or develop instruments for collecting data	4.3.2 4.3.3 4.3.4 4.3.5 4.3.6	Adapt/modify existing data collection instruments Create new data collection instruments Identify useable items from existing instruments Adapt/modify existing items Create new items to be used in data collection		

Appendix B.2: Comparison of the Competencies and Sub-competencies of the HESPA II 2020 Model to the HESPA I 2015 Model

Key: Entry level = No symbol; Advanced-1 (▲); Advanced-2 (■)
  Sub-competency worded the same in both Frameworks is indicated under comments

HESPA II Code	HESPA II 2020	HESPA I Code	HESPA I 2015	Comments
	Area IV: Evaluation and Research			**Comments**
4.2.9 ■	Implement a pilot test to refine and validate data collection instruments and procedures	4.3.7 4.3.8 4.3.9 4.3.10 ■	Pilot test data collection instrument Establish validity of data collection instruments Ensure that data collection instruments generate reliable data Ensure fairness of data collection instruments (for example, reduce bias, use language appropriate to priority population)	
4.3	**Manage the collection and analysis of evaluation and/or research data using appropriate technology**	**4.4**	**Collect and manage data**	
4.3.1 ■	Train data collectors	1.3.4 4.4.1	Train personnel assisting with data collection Train data collectors involved in evaluation and/or research	
4.3.2	Implement data collection procedures	1.3.5 4.4.2	Implement quantitative and/or qualitative data collection Collect data based on the evaluation or research plan	
4.3.3	Use appropriate modalities to collect and manage data	4.4.3 4.4.4	Monitor and manage data collection. Use available technology to collect, monitor and manage data	
4.3.4 ■	Monitor data collection procedures	4.4.3	Monitor and manage data collection	
4.3.5	Prepare data for analysis	4.5.1	Prepare data for analysis	Same wording
4.3.6 ■	Analyze data	4.5.2 4.5.3 4.5.4 4.5.5	Analyze data using qualitative methods Analyze data using descriptive statistical methods Analyze data using inferential statistical methods Use technology to analyze data	

Appendix B.2: Comparison of the Competencies and Sub-competencies of the HESPA II 2020 Model to the HESPA I 2015 Model

Key: Entry level = No symbol; Advanced-1 (▲); Advanced-2 (■)
Sub-competency worded the same in both Frameworks is indicated under comments

HESPA II Code	HESPA II 2020	HESPA I Code	HESPA I 2015	
	Area IV: Evaluation and Research			**Comments**
4.4	**Interpret data**	**4.5** **4.6**	**Analyze data** **Interpret results**	
4.4.1 ■	Explain how findings address the questions and/or hypotheses	4.6.1 4.6.2	Synthesize the analyzed data Explain how the results address the questions and/or hypotheses	
4.4.2 ▲	Compare findings to other evaluations or studies	4.6.3	Compare findings to results from other studies or evaluations	
4.4.3	Identify limitations and delimitations of findings	4.6.5 4.6.6	Identify limitations of findings Address delimitations as they relate to findings	
4.4.4 ■	Draw conclusions based on findings	4.6.7	Draw conclusions based on findings	Same Wording
4.4.5 ■	Identify implications for practice			No match
4.4.6 ■	Synthesize findings	4.6.1 4.6.4	Synthesize the analyzed data Propose possible explanations for findings	
4.4.7 ■	Develop recommendations based on findings	4.6.8	Develop recommendations based on findings	Same wording
4.4.8 ■	Evaluate feasibility of implementing recommendations	4.7.3	Evaluate feasibility of implementing recommendations	Same wording
4.5	**Use findings**	**4.7**	**Apply findings**	
4.5.1 ▲	Communicate findings by preparing reports and presentations, and by other means	4.7.1	Communicate findings to priority populations, partners, and stakeholders	
4.5.2 ■	Disseminate findings	4.7.5	Disseminate findings using a variety of methods	
4.5.3 ■	Identify recommendations for quality improvement	4.6.8 ■ 4.7.4	Develop recommendations based on findings Incorporate findings into program improvement and refinement	

Appendix B.2: Comparison of the Competencies and Sub-competencies of the HESPA II 2020 Model to the HESPA I 2015 Model

Key: Entry level = No symbol; Advanced-1 (▲); Advanced-2 (■)
Sub-competency worded the same in both Frameworks is indicated under comments

HESPA II Code	HESPA II 2020	HESPA I Code	HESPA I 2015	
	Area IV: Evaluation and Research			**Comments**
4.5.4 ▲	Translate findings into practice and interventions	4.6.8 ■ 4.7.4	Develop recommendations based on findings Incorporate findings into program improvement and refinement	
	Area V: Advocacy			**Comments**
5.1	**Identify a current or emerging health issue requiring policy, systems, or environmental change**			
5.1.1	Examine the determinants of health and their underlying causes (e.g., poverty, trauma, and population-based discrimination) related to identified health issues	1.4.1 1.4.2 1.4.3 7.2.1	Identify and analyze factors that influence health behaviors Identify and analyze factors that impact health Identify the impact of emerging social, economic, and other trends on health Identify current and emerging issues requiring advocacy	
5.1.2	Examine evidence-informed findings related to identified health issues and desired changes	1.2.5 7.2.1 7.3.5	Extract data from existing databases. Identify current and emerging issues requiring advocacy Use evidence-based findings in policy analysis	
5.1.3	Identify factors that facilitate and/or hinder advocacy efforts (e.g., amount of evidence to prove the issue, potential for partnerships, political readiness, organizational experience or risk, and feasibility of success)			No match
5.1.4	Write specific, measurable, achievable, realistic, and time-bound (SMART) advocacy objective(s)	2.2.5	Develop specific, measurable, attainable, realistic, and time-sensitive objectives	
5.1.5	Identify existing coalition(s) or stakeholders that can be engaged in advocacy efforts	2.1.1 7.2.2	Identify priority populations, partners, and other stakeholders Engage stakeholders in advocacy initiatives	

Appendix B.2: Comparison of the Competencies and Sub-competencies of the HESPA II 2020 Model to the HESPA I 2015 Model

Key: Entry level = No symbol; Advanced-1 (▲); Advanced-2 (■)
Sub-competency worded the same in both Frameworks is indicated under comments

HESPA II Code	HESPA II 2020	HESPA I Code	HESPA I 2015	
	Area V: Advocacy			**Comments**
5.2	**Engage coalitions and stakeholders in addressing the health issue and planning advocacy efforts**			
5.2.1	Identify existing coalitions and stakeholders that favor and oppose the proposed policy, system, or environmental change and their reasons			No match
5.2.2	Identify factors that influence decision-makers (e.g., societal and cultural norms, financial considerations, upcoming elections, and voting record)	7.3.7	Identify factors that influence decision-makers	
5.2.3 ▲	Create formal and/or informal alliances, task forces, and coalitions to address the proposed change	7.2.2 7.2.9	Engage stakeholders in advocacy initiatives Lead advocacy initiatives related to health	
5.2.4	Educate stakeholders on the health issue and the proposed policy, system, or environmental change	7.2.2 7.3.8	Engage stakeholders in advocacy initiatives Use policy advocacy techniques to influence decision-makers	
5.2.5	Identify available resources and gaps (e.g., financial, personnel, information, and data)	7.2.3	Access resources (for example, financial, personnel, information, data) related to identified advocacy needs	
5.2.6	Identify organizational policies and procedures and federal, state, and local laws that pertain to the advocacy efforts	7.2.4	Develop advocacy plans in compliance with local, state, and/or federal policies and procedures	
5.2.7	Develop persuasive messages and materials (e.g., briefs, resolutions, and fact sheets) to communicate the policy, system, or environmental change	3.1.2 7.2.5 7.3.4 7.3.8	Develop materials to implement plan Use strategies that advance advocacy goals Project the impact of proposed systems changes on health education Use policy advocacy techniques to influence decision-makers	

Appendix B.2: Comparison of the Competencies and Sub-competencies of the HESPA II 2020 Model to the HESPA I 2015 Model

Key: Entry level = No symbol; Advanced-1 (▲); Advanced-2 (■)

Sub-competency worded the same in both Frameworks is indicated under comments

HESPA II Code	HESPA II 2020	HESPA I Code	HESPA I 2015	Comments
	Area V: Advocacy			**Comments**
5.2.8	Specify strategies, a timeline, and roles and responsibilities to address the proposed policy, system, or environmental change (e.g., develop ongoing relationships with decision makers and stakeholders, use social media, register others to vote, and seek political appointment)	7.2.5 7.2.9 7.3.8	Use strategies that advance advocacy goals Lead advocacy initiatives related to health Use policy advocacy techniques to influence decision-makers	
5.3	**Engage in advocacy**			
5.3.1	Use media to conduct advocacy (e.g., social media, press releases, public service announcements, and op-eds)	7.2.5 7.3.9	Use strategies that advance advocacy goals Use media advocacy techniques to influence decision-makers	
5.3.2	Use traditional, social, and emerging technologies and methods to mobilize support for policy, system, or environmental change	7.2.5 7.2.6 7.3.8 7.3.10	Use strategies that advance advocacy goals Implement advocacy plans Use policy advocacy techniques to influence decision-makers Engage in legislative advocacy	
5.3.3 ▲	Sustain coalitions and stakeholder relationships to achieve and maintain policy, system, or environmental change	7.2.5 7.2.6 7.3.8	Use strategies that advance advocacy goals Implement advocacy plans Use policy advocacy techniques to influence decision-makers	
5.4	**Evaluate advocacy**			**Comments**
5.4.1	Conduct process, impact, and outcome evaluation of advocacy efforts	7.2.7	Evaluate advocacy efforts	
5.4.2	Use the results of the evaluation to inform next steps			No match
	Area VI: Communication			**Comments**
6.1	**Determine factors that affect communication with the identified audience(s)**			
6.1.1	Segment the audience(s) to be addressed, as needed			No match

Appendix B.2: Comparison of the Competencies and Sub-competencies of the HESPA II 2020 Model to the HESPA I 2015 Model

Key: Entry level = No symbol; Advanced-1 (▲); Advanced-2 (■)

Sub-competency worded the same in both Frameworks is indicated under comments

HESPA II Code	HESPA II 2020	HESPA I Code	HESPA I 2015	Comments
	Area VI: Communication			**Comments**
6.1.2	Identify the assets, needs, and characteristics of the audience(s) that affect communication and message design (e.g., literacy levels, language, culture, and cognitive and perceptual abilities)	6.1.1 / 7.1.2	Assess needs for health-related information / Identify level of literacy of intended audience	
6.1.3	Identify communication channels (e.g., social media and mass media) available to and used by the audience(s)	2.4.6 / 7.1.6	Select methods and/or channels for reaching priority populations / Assess and select methods and technologies used to deliver messages	
6.1.4	Identify environmental and other factors that affect communication (e.g., resources and the availability of Internet access)	1.6.4	Assess social, environmental, political, and other factors that may impact health education/promotion	
6.2	**Determine communication objective(s) for audience(s)**			
6.2.1	Describe the intended outcome of the communication (e.g., raise awareness, advocacy, behavioral change, and risk communication)	2.2.1	Identify desired outcomes using the needs assessment results	
6.2.2	Write specific, measurable, achievable, realistic, and time-bound (SMART) communication objective(s)	2.2.5	Develop specific, measurable, attainable, realistic, and time-sensitive objectives	
6.2.3	Identify factors that facilitate and/or hinder the intended outcome of the communication	1.6.4	Assess social, environmental, political, and other factors that may impact health education/promotion	
6.3	**Develop message(s) using communication theories and/or models**			
6.3.1	Use communications theory to develop or select communication message(s)	7.1.1	Create messages using communication theories and/or models	
6.3.2	Develop persuasive communications (e.g., storytelling and program rationale)	5.4.4	Use various communication strategies to present rationale	
6.3.3	Tailor message(s) for the audience(s)	6.1.4 / 7.1.3	Adapt information for consumer / Tailor messages for intended audience	Same wording

Appendix B.2: Comparison of the Competencies and Sub-competencies of the HESPA II 2020 Model to the HESPA I 2015 Model

Key: Entry level = No symbol; Advanced-1 (▲); Advanced-2 (■)
   Sub-competency worded the same in both Frameworks is indicated under comments

HESPA II Code	HESPA II 2020	HESPA I Code	HESPA I 2015	Comments
	Area VI: Communication			**Comments**
6.3.4	Employ media literacy skills (e.g., identifying credible sources and balancing multiple viewpoints)			No match
6.4	**Select methods and technologies used to deliver message(s)**			
6.4.1	Differentiate the strengths and weaknesses of various communication channels and technologies (e.g., mass media, community mobilization, counseling, peer communication, information/digital technology, and apps)	7.1.6	Assess and select methods and technologies used to deliver messages	
6.4.2	Select communication channels and current and emerging technologies that are most appropriate for the audience(s) and message(s)	7.1.6 / 7.1.7	Assess and select methods and technologies used to deliver messages / Deliver messages using media and communication strategies	
6.4.3	Develop communication aids, materials, or tools using appropriate multimedia (e.g., infographics, presentation software, brochures, and posters)	3.1.2	Develop materials to implement plan	
6.4.4	Assess the suitability of new and/or existing communication aids, materials, or tools for audience(s) (e.g., the CDC Clear Communication Index and the Suitability Assessment of Materials [SAM])	6.1.3 / 7.1.6	Evaluate resource materials for accuracy, relevance, and timeliness / Assess and select methods and technologies used to deliver messages	
6.4.5	Pilot test message(s) and communication aids, materials, or tools	7.1.4	Pilot test messages and delivery methods	
6.4.6	Revise communication aids, materials, or tools based on pilot results	7.1.5	Revise messages based on pilot feedback	
6.5	**Deliver the message(s) effectively using the identified media and strategies**			
6.5.1	Deliver presentation(s) tailored to the audience(s)	6.1.5 / 7.1.7	Convey health-related information to consumer / Deliver messages using media and communication strategies	

Appendix B.2: Comparison of the Competencies and Sub-competencies of the HESPA II 2020 Model to the HESPA I 2015 Model

Key: Entry level = No symbol; Advanced-1 (▲); Advanced-2 (■)
Sub-competency worded the same in both Frameworks is indicated under comments

HESPA II Code	HESPA II 2020	HESPA I Code	HESPA I 2015	
	Area VI: Communication			**Comments**
6.5.2	Use public speaking skills			No match
6.5.3	Use facilitation skills with large and/or small groups			No match
6.5.4	Use current and emerging communication tools and trends (e.g., social media)	7.1.7	Deliver messages using media and communication strategies	
6.5.5	Deliver oral and written communication that aligns with professional standards of grammar, punctuation, and style	6.1.5 7.1.7	Convey health-related information to consumer Deliver messages using media and communication strategies	
6.5.6	Use digital media to engage audience(s) (e.g., social media management tools and platforms)	7.1.7	Deliver messages using media and communication strategies	
6.6	**Evaluate communication**			
6.6.1	Conduct process and impact evaluations of communications			
6.6.2 ■	Conduct outcome evaluations of communications	7.1.7	Deliver messages using media and communication strategies	
6.6.3 ▲	Assess reach and dose of communication using tools (e.g., data mining software, social media analytics, and website analytics)	7.1.8	Evaluate the impact of the delivered messages	
	Area VII: Leadership and Management			**Comments**
7.1	**Coordinate relationships with partners and stakeholders (e.g. individuals, teams, coalitions, and committees)**	**5.3**	**Manage financial resources for health education/promotion programs**	
7.1.1	Identify potential partners and stakeholders	2.1.1	Identify priority populations, partners, and other stakeholders	
7.1.2	Assess the capacity of potential partners and stakeholders	5.3.1	Assess capacity of partners and other stakeholders to meet program goals	

Appendix B.2: Comparison of the Competencies and Sub-competencies of the HESPA II 2020 Model to the HESPA I 2015 Model

Key: Entry level = No symbol; Advanced-1 (▲); Advanced-2 (■)
Sub-competency worded the same in both Frameworks is indicated under comments

HESPA II Code	HESPA II 2020	HESPA I Code	HESPA I 2015	Comments
	Area VII: Leadership and Management			
7.1.3	Involve partners and stakeholders throughout the health education and promotion process in meaningful and sustainable ways	5.3.2 5.3.5 ▲	Facilitate discussions with partners and other stakeholders regarding program resource needs Elicit feedback from partners and other stakeholders	
7.1.4 ▲	Execute formal and informal agreements with partners and stakeholders	2.1.5 5.3.3	Obtain commitments to participate in health education/promotion Elicit feedback from partners and other stakeholders	
7.1.5	Evaluate relationships with partners and stakeholders on an ongoing basis to make appropriate modifications	5.3.4 5.3.5 ▲ 5.3.6	Monitor relationships with partners and other stakeholders Elicit feedback from partners and other stakeholders Evaluate relationships with partners and other stakeholders	
7.2	**Prepare others to provide health education and promotion**	**6.2**	**Train others to use health education/ promotion skills**	
7.2.1	Develop culturally responsive content	3.3.4	Apply principles of diversity and cultural competence in implementing health education/promotion plan	
7.2.2	Recruit individuals needed in implementation	3.2.2 5.6.5	Recruit individuals needed for implementation Recruit staff members and volunteers for programs	Same wording
7.2.3 ▲	Assess training needs	3.2.3 6.2.1	Identify training needs of individuals involved in implementation Assess training needs of potential participants	
7.2.4 ▲	Plan training, including technical assistance and support	3.2.4 3.2.6 6.2.2 6.2.3	Develop training using best practices Provide support and technical assistance to those implementing the plan Develop a plan for conducting training Identify resources needed to conduct training	

Appendix B.2: Comparison of the Competencies and Sub-competencies of the HESPA II 2020 Model to the HESPA I 2015 Model

Key: Entry level = No symbol; Advanced-1 (▲); Advanced-2 (■)
Sub-competency worded the same in both Frameworks is indicated under comments

HESPA II Code	HESPA II 2020	HESPA I Code	HESPA I 2015	Comments
	Area VII: Leadership and Management			Comments
7.2.5 ▲	Implement training	3.2.5 6.2.4	Implement training Implement planned training	Same wording
7.2.6 ▲	Evaluate training as appropriate throughout the process	3.2.7 6.2.5 6.2.6	Evaluate training Conduct formative and summative evaluations of training Use evaluative feedback to create future trainings	
7.3	**Manage human resources**	**5.6**	**Manage human resources for health education/promotion programs**	
7.3.1 ▲	Facilitate understanding and sensitivity for various cultures, values, and traditions	3.3.4	Apply principles of diversity and cultural competence in implementing health education/promotion plan	
7.3.2 ▲	Facilitate positive organizational culture and climate	5.5.2 5.5.3 5.5.4	Analyze an organization's culture to determine the extent to which it supports health education/promotion Develop strategies to reinforce or change organizational culture to support health education/promotion Facilitate needed changes to organizational culture	
7.3.3 ▲	Develop job descriptions to meet staffing needs	5.6.2 5.6.4.	Develop job descriptions Evaluate qualifications of staff members and volunteers needed for program	
7.3.4 ▲	Recruit qualified staff (including paraprofessionals) and volunteers	5.6.5	Recruit staff members and volunteers for programs	
7.3.5 ▲	Evaluate performance of staff and volunteers formally and informally	5.6.6 ▲ 5.6.12	Determine staff member and volunteer professional development needs Evaluate performance of staff members and volunteers	
7.3.6 ▲	Provide professional development and training for staff and volunteers	5.6.7 5.6.8	Develop strategies to enhance staff member and volunteer professional development Implement strategies to enhance the professional development of staff members and volunteers	

Appendix B.2: Comparison of the Competencies and Sub-competencies of the HESPA II 2020 Model to the HESPA I 2015 Model

Key: Entry level = No symbol; Advanced-1 (▲); Advanced-2 (■)
  Sub-competency worded the same in both Frameworks is indicated under comments

HESPA II Code	HESPA II 2020	HESPA I Code	HESPA I 2015	Comments
	Area VII: Leadership and Management			**Comments**
7.3.7 ▲	Facilitate the engagement and retention of staff and volunteers	5.6.9	Develop and implement strategies to retain staff members and volunteers	
7.3.8 ▲	Apply team building and conflict resolution techniques as appropriate	5.6.10 5.6.11	Employ conflict resolution techniques Facilitate team development	
7.4	**Manage fiduciary and material resources**	**5.1**	**Manage financial resources for health education/promotion**	
7.4.1 ▲	Evaluate internal and external financial needs and funding sources	5.1.2 5.1.3	Evaluate financial needs and resources Identify internal and/or external funding sources	
7.4.2 ▲	Develop financial budgets and plans	5.1.1 5.1.5	Develop financial plan Develop program budgets	
7.4.3 ▲	Monitor budget performance	5.1.6 5.1.9	Manage program budgets Monitor financial plan	
7.4.4 ■	Justify value of health education and promotion using economic (e.g., cost-benefit, return-on-investment, and value-on-investment) and/or other analyses	5.1.7 5.4.2 5.4.3	Conduct cost analysis for programs Identify evidence to justify programs Create a rationale to gain or maintain program support	
7.4.5 ▲	Write grants and funding proposals	5.1.10 5.1.11	Create requests for funding proposals Write grant proposals	
7.4.6 ■	Conduct reviews of funding and grant proposals	5.1.12	Conduct reviews of funding proposals	
7.4.7 ▲	Monitor performance and/or compliance of funding recipients	5.6.13	Monitor performance and/or compliance of funding recipients	Same wording
7.4.8 ▲	Maintain up-to-date technology infrastructure	5.2.2 5.2.4	Use technology to collect, store and retrieve program management data Evaluate emerging technologies for applicability to health education/promotion	
7.4.9 ▲	Manage current and future facilities and resources (e.g., space and equipment)			No match

Appendix B.2: Comparison of the Competencies and Sub-competencies of the HESPA II 2020 Model to the HESPA I 2015 Model

Key: Entry level = No symbol; Advanced-1 (▲); Advanced-2 (■)
Sub-competency worded the same in both Frameworks is indicated under comments

HESPA II Code	HESPA II 2020	HESPA I Code	HESPA I 2015	
	Area VII: Leadership and Management			**Comments**
7.5	**Conduct strategic planning with appropriate stakeholders**	**5.5**	**Demonstrate leadership**	
7.5.1 ▲	Facilitate the development of strategic and/or improvement plans using systems thinking to promote the mission, vision, and goal statements for health education and promotion	5.5.1 5.5.4 5.5.5	Facilitate efforts to achieve organizational mission Facilitate needed changes to organizational structure Conduct strategic planning	
7.5.2 ▲	Gain organizational acceptance for strategic and/or improvement plans	5.5.3	Develop strategies to reinforce or change organizational culture to support health education/promotion	
7.5.3 ▲	Implement the strategic plan, incorporating status updates and making refinements as appropriate	5.5.6 5.5.7 5.5.8	Implement strategic plan Monitor strategic plan Conduct program quality assurance/process improvement	
	Area VIII: Ethics and Professionalism			**Comments**
8.1	**Practice in accordance with established ethical principles**			
8.1.1	Apply professional codes of ethics and ethical principles throughout assessment, planning, implementation, evaluation and research, communication, consulting, and advocacy processes (continued on page 159)	1.1.5 2.3.11 3.1.5 3.4.8 4.1.10 4.2.14 4.3.10 5.1.13 5.2.3	Apply ethical principles to the assessment process Apply ethical principles in selecting strategies and designing interventions Apply ethical principles to the implementation process Monitor adherence to ethical principles in the implementation of health education/promotion Apply ethical principles to the evaluation process Apply ethical principles to the research process Ensure fairness of data collection instruments (for example, reduce bias, use language appropriate to priority population) Apply ethical principles when managing financial resources Apply ethical principles in managing technology resources	

Appendix B.2: Comparison of the Competencies and Sub-competencies of the HESPA II 2020 Model to the HESPA I 2015 Model

Key: Entry level = No symbol; Advanced-1 (▲); Advanced-2 (■)

Sub-competency worded the same in both Frameworks is indicated under comments

	HESPA II 2020	HESPA I Code	HESPA I 2015		
	Area VIII: Ethics and Professionalism				**Comments**
8.1.1	Apply professional codes of ethics and ethical principles throughout assessment, planning, implementation, evaluation and research, communication, consulting, and advocacy processes (continued from page 158)	5.5.10 5.6.14 6.3.5	Adhere to ethical principles of the profession Apply ethical principles when managing human resources Apply ethical principles in consultative relationships		
8.1.2 ▲	Demonstrate ethical leadership, management, and behavior				
8.1.3	Comply with legal standards and regulatory guidelines in assessment, planning, implementation, evaluation and research, advocacy, management, communication, and reporting processes	2.3.12 3.1.6 3.4.7 4.4.5 5.5.9 5.6.3 7.2.4 7.2.8	Comply with legal standards in selecting strategies and designing interventions Comply with legal standards that apply to implementation Ensure compliance with legal standards Comply with laws and regulations when collecting, storing, and protecting participant data Comply with existing laws and regulations Apply human resource policies consistent with laws and regulations Develop advocacy plans in compliance with local, state, and/or federal policies and procedures Comply with organizational policies related to participating in advocacy		
8.1.4	Promote health equity				No match
8.1.5	Use evidence-informed theories, models, and strategies	1.1.4 2.3.3 2.4.1 3.2.4 ▲ 3.3.2 7.1.1 7.3.6 ▲	Apply theories and/or models to assessment process Apply principles of evidence-based practice in selecting and/or designing strategies/interventions Use theories and/or models to guide the delivery plan Develop training using best practices Apply theories and/or models of implementation Create messages using communication theories and/or models Develop policies to promote health using evidence-based findings		

Appendix B.2: Comparison of the Competencies and Sub-competencies of the HESPA II 2020 Model to the HESPA I 2015 Model

Key: Entry level = No symbol; Advanced-1 (▲); Advanced-2 (■)
   Sub-competency worded the same in both Frameworks is indicated under comments

HESPA II Code	HESPA II 2020	HESPA I Code	HESPA I 2015	Comments
	Area VIII: Ethics and Professionalism			
8.1.6	Apply principles of cultural humility, inclusion, and diversity in all aspects of practice (e.g., Culturally and Linguistically Appropriate Services (CLAS) standards and culturally responsive pedagogy)	2.3.4 2.3.5 3.3.4 4.3.10	Apply principles of cultural competence in selecting and/or designing strategies/interventions Address diversity within priority populations in selecting and/or designing strategies/interventions Apply principles of diversity and cultural competence in implementing health education/promotion plan Ensure fairness of data collection instruments (for example, reduce bias, use language appropriate to priority population)	
8.2	**Serve as an authoritative resource on health education and promotion**	**6.3**	**Provide advice and consultation on health education/promotion issues**	
8.2.1 ▲	Evaluate personal and organizational capacity to provide consultation	6.3.1	Assess and prioritize requests for advice/consultation	
8.2.2 ▲	Provide expert consultation, assistance, and guidance to individuals, groups, and organizations	6.3.3	Provide expert assistance and guidance	
8.2.3 ■	Conduct peer reviews (e.g., manuscripts, abstracts, proposals, and tenure folios)	6.3.3 7.4.11	Provide expert assistance and guidance Engage in service to advance the profession	
8.3	**Engage in professional development to maintain and/or enhance proficiency**			
8.3.1	Participate in professional associations, coalitions, and networks (e.g., serving on committees, attending conferences, and providing leadership)	7.4.8 7.4.11	Develop and implement a professional development plan Engage in service to advance the profession	
8.3.2	Participate in continuing education opportunities to maintain or enhance continuing competence	7.4.8	Develop and implement a professional development plan	
8.3.3	Develop a career advancement plan	7.4.8	Develop and implement a professional development plan	

Appendix B.2: Comparison of the Competencies and Sub-competencies of the HESPA II 2020 Model to the HESPA I 2015 Model

Key: Entry level = No symbol; Advanced-1 (▲); Advanced-2 (■)
Sub-competency worded the same in both Frameworks is indicated under comments

HESPA II Code	HESPA II 2020	HESPA I Code	HESPA I 2015	Comments
	Area VIII: Ethics and Professionalism			**Comments**
8.3.4	Build relationships with other professionals within and outside the profession	6.3.2 ▲	Establish advisory/consultative relationships	
8.3.5 ■	Serve as a mentor	7.4.9	Serve as a mentor to others in the profession	
8.4	**Promote the health education profession to stakeholders, the public, and others**	**7.4**	**Promote the health education profession**	
8.4.1	Explain the major responsibilities, contributions, and value of the health education specialist	7.4.1	Explain the major responsibilities of the health education specialist	
8.4.2	Explain the role of professional organizations and the benefits of participating in them	7.4.2 7.4.3	Explain the role of professional organizations in advancing the profession Explain the benefits of participating in professional organizations	
8.4.3	Advocate for professional development for health education specialists	7.4.4 7.4.5	Advocate for professional development of health education specialists Advocate for the profession	Same wording
8.4.4	Educate others about the history of the profession, its current status, and its implications for professional practice	7.4.5 7.4.6	Advocate for the profession Explain the history of the profession and its current and future implications for professional practice	
8.4.5	Explain the role and benefits of credentialing (e.g., individual and program)	7.4.7	Explain the role of credentialing (for example, individual, program) in the promotion of the profession	
8.4.6 ▲	Develop presentations and publications that contribute to the profession	7.4.10	Develop materials that contribute to the professional literature	
8.4.7 ▲	Engage in service to advance the profession	7.4.11	Engage in service to advance the profession	Same wording

Appendix B.2: Comparison of the Competencies and Sub-competencies of the HESPA II 2020 Model to the HESPA I 2015 Model

Notes:

Appendix C: History of Working Groups for Health Education Specialist Competency Development

The list of Committees, Task Forces and other working groups who contributed to the Health Education Specialist Practice Analysis II (HESPA II 2020) is provided below. The various committees and other working groups who contributed to the Health Education Specialist Practice Analysis I (HESPA I 2015), the Health Educator Job Analysis (HEJA 2010), the Competencies Update Project (CUP) and previous committees who worked on defining the role and Competencies of the health education profession are also listed.

Health Education Specialist Practice Analysis II 2020 (HESPA II 2020): 2017-2019

Scantron Assessment Solutions Inc.
James Henderson, Ph.D.

HESPA II 2020 Technical Advisory Group (TAG)
Randall R. Cottrell, D.Ed., MCHES® (Chair)
Adam P. Knowlden, MBA, Ph.D., CHES® (Vice -Chair)
Kathleen Allison, Ph.D., MPH, MCHES®
M. Elaine Auld, MPH, MCHES®
James F. McKenzie, Ph.D., MPH, MCHES®
Linda Lysoby, MS, MCHES®, CAE
Cynthia S. Kusorgbor-Narh, MPH, MCHES®

HESPA II 2020 Health Education Practice Panel (HEPP)
Sue M. Baldwin, MEd, Ph.D., MCHES®, FASHA
Radhika Bhavsar, MPH, CHES®
David A. Birch, Ph.D., MCHES®
Mario C. Browne, MPH, CHES®, CDP
Melissa Cordeiro, BS, CHES®
Bridget A. Cross, MA, CHES®
Amanda Greene, RN, BSN, MCHES®
Chandra Alise Jennings, Ph.D., MSE, CHES®
Sarojini Kanotra, Ph.D., MPH, CHES®
Cynthia Karlsson, MPH, MS, CHES®
Suzanne Lineberry, MPH, MCHES®
Elisa "Beth" McNeill, Ph.D., CHES®
Kate Muskrat, MS
Cherylee Sherry, MPH, MCHES®
Michael J. Staufacker, MA, MCHES®
Jila M. Tanha, MPH, CHES®
Jennifer Torres, MPH, CHES®

HESPA II 2020 Pilot Test Participants
Laura Chandler, DrPH, MCHES®
Beth Chaney, Ph.D., MCHES®
Jesseca Chatman, MPH, CHES®
Meifang Chen, Ph.D., MCHES®
Dixie Dennis, Ph.D., MCHES®, FAAHE
Ashley Glass, MPH, CHES®
Brandon Horvath, MPH
Chandra Jennings-Jackson, BS, CHES®
Kathy Jinkins, BSN, M.Ed., MCHES®
Dianne Kerr, Ph.D., MCHES®
David Lohrmann, Ph.D., MCHES®
Renee Ann Mallari, BS, CHES®
Jennifer Morel, MPH, CHES®
Julie Reeder, Ph.D., CHES®
Kathleen Riley, MPH, CHES®
Doreleena Sammons Hackett, MS
Amy Sidwell, Ph.D., CHES®
LT. Tanesha G. Tutt, Ph.D., CHES®
Robin Vlamis, MPH, CHES®
Teresa Marie Vogt, MEd, CHES®

Health Education Specialist Practice Analysis I 2015 (HESPA I 2015): 2013-2014

Professional Examination Service
Carla M. Caro, MA
Patricia M. Muenzen, MA
Dianne Henderson-Montero, Ph.D.

NCHEC Support Staff
Cynthia S. Kusorgbor-Narh, MPH, CHES

Note: Trademark for the CHES® and MCHES® credentials officially registered with the United States Patent and Trademark Office in 2017

Appendix C: History of Working Groups for Health Education Specialist Competency Development

HESPA I 2015 Steering Committee
M. Elaine Auld, MPH, MCHES
Dixie Dennis, Ph.D., MCHES
Eva I. Doyle, Ph.D., MSEd, MCHES
Linda Lysoby, MS, MCHES, CAE
James F. McKenzie, Ph.D., MPH, MCHES

HESPA I 2015 Task Force
Dixie Dennis, Ph.D., MCHES (Co-chair)
James F. McKenzie, Ph.D., MPH, MCHES (Co-chair)
Kelly Brennan, MEd, MCHES
Annie L. Dickerson, MA, CHES
Michele Guadalupe, MPH
Gilberto Hernandez, MA, CHES
Michael Staufacker, MA, MCHES
Grace Salako Smith, Ph.D., CHES
Alyson Taub, Ph.D., MCHES
Linh Tran, BS, CHES
Starr Wharton, MS, MCHES
Alexis Williams, MPH, CHES

HESPA I 2015 Telephone Interview Panel
David Birch, Ph.D., MCHES
Karen Cottrell, MEd
Gary D. Gilmore, Ph.D., MPH, MCHES
Susan Goekler, Ph.D., MCHES
Madonna Lynn Holbrook-Lowe, MPH, MCHES
Garry M. Lindsay, MPH, MCHES
Michael McNeil, MS, Ed.D, CHES
Sarah J. Olson, MS, CHES
Dan Perales, DrPH, MPH
Susan M. Radius, PhD, MCHES
Robert F. Valois MS, PhD, MPH, FAAHB

HESPA I 2015 Independent Review Panel
Christine Abarca, MPH, MCHES
Leititia Bailey, MPH, CHES
Srijana M. Bajrachrya, Ph.D., MCHES
Mario C. Browne, MPH, CHES
Brenda Carter
Blanche Collins, MHSE, MCHES

Sonja Davis, BS, CHES
Bonnie J. Edmondson, Ed.D, MS
Richard Edwards, PhD, CHES
Jim Grizzell, MA, MBA, MCHES
Stacy Haitsuka, MPH, CHES
Maureen W. Krouse, BS, CHES
Teresa Lovely, MS, MCHES
Carol Noel Michaels, MPH, MCHES
Chanita W. Neal, MHSE, CHES
Larry Olsen, DrPH, MCHES
Patricia G. Owen, MCHES
Tamara Oyola-Santiago, MPH, CHES
Carrie Shult, MHS, CHES
Robert Walker, Ph.D., MS

HESPA I 2015 Pilot Test Participants
David Brown, Ed.D, MCHES
Yyolany Caffrey, MPH, CHES
Lisa Clough, MSEd, CHES
Emily Dunnebacke, BS, CHES
Jody Early, Ph.D., MCHES
Amanda Graves, BSEd, CHES
Jake Hanson, BS, CHES
Patty Holman, MS, CHES
Katie Jourdan, MPH, CHES
Sarojini Kanotra, Ph.D, CHES
Emily Lee, MEd, CHES
Lindsey Mitchell, MPH
Charlotte Petonic, BS, CHES
Janet Pryor, BS
Estelle Raboni, MPH, CHES
Krista Reale, MA, CHES
Patti Rittling, Ph.D., CHES
Keiko Sakagami, Ed.D, MCHES
Kimberley Sinclair, MPH
Caile Spear, Ph.D, MCHES
Chelsea Stone, BS, CHES
Jerah Thomas, MPH, CHES
Chantay Williams, MPH
Holly Wilson, MHSE, CHES

Appendix C: History of Working Groups for Health Education Specialist Competency Development

Authors and Editors of *A Competency-Based Framework for Health Education Specialists – 2015*

James F. McKenzie, PhD, MPH, MCHES
Dixie Dennis, PhD, MCHES
Kelly Brennan, MEd, MCHES
Randall Cottrell, DEd, MCHES
Eva I Doyle, PhD, MCHES
Jenni Flanagan, BS, CHES
Michele Guadalupe, MPH
Cynthia S. Kusorgbor-Narh, MPH, CHES
Denise M. Seabert, PhD, MCHES
Starr Wharton, MS, MCHES
Caitlin Rizzo, MS

National Health Educator Job Analysis 2010 (HEJA 2010): 2008-2009

Professional Examination Service
Carla M. Caro, MA
Patricia M. Muenzen, MA

HEJA 2010 Steering Committee
M. Elaine Auld, MPH, CHES
Eva I. Doyle, PhD, MSEd, CHES
Linda Lysoby, MS, CHES, CAE
Beverly Saxton Mahoney, RN, MS, PhD, CHES
Becky J. Smith, PhD, CHES, CAE

HEJA 2010 Task Force
Eva I. Doyle, PhD, MSEd, CHES (Chair)
Kelly Bishop Alley, MA, CHES
Chesley Cheatham, MEd, CHES
Lillie M. Hall, MPH, CHES
Mary Marks, PhD
James F. McKenzie, PhD, MPH, CHES
Michael P. McNeil, MS, CHES
Darcy Scharff, PhD
Michael Staufacker, MA, CHES
Alyson Taub, PhD, CHES
Carol A. Younkin, RN, MA, CHES

HEJA 2010 Telephone Interview Panel
John Allegrante, PhD
Nancy Atmospera-Walch, RN, BSN, MPH, CHES
Karen Cottrell, MEd
Gary Gilmore, PhD, MPH, CHES
James Grizzell, MA, MBA, CHES
Pamela Hoalt, PhD, LPC
Jacqueline Valenzuela, MPH, CHES
Louise Villejo, MPH, CHES
C. Lynn Woodhouse, EdD, MPH

HEJA 2010 Independent Review Panel
Edith Cabuslay, MPH
Elizabeth H. Chaney, PhD, CHES
Dixie L. Dennis, PhD, CHES
Marcy Harrington, MPA, CHES
Jon W. Hisgen, MS, CHES
Judith A. Johns, MS, CHES
Linda LaSalle, PhD
Garry M. Lindsay, MPH, CHES
Kimberley McBride, MPH
Larry K. Olsen, DrPH, CHES
Deyonne M. Sandoval, MS, CHES
Audrey E. Shively, MSHSE, CHES
Rob Simmons, DrPH, MPH, CHES
Cortney E. Smith, MS, CHES
Virginia Smyly, MPH, CHES
Francisco Soto Mas, MD, PhD, MPH
Jody R. Steinhardt, MPH, CHES

HEJA 2010 Pilot Test Participants
Dori Babcock, MA
Janet Baggett, MA, CHES
Christine E. Beyer, PhD
Johanna Chase, MA, CHES
Chia-Ching Chen, EdD, CHES
Lori Elmore, MPH, CHES
Brian F. Geiger, PhD
Amanda Greene, PhD, CHES
Harpreet Grewal, MPH, CHES

Appendix C: History of Working Groups for Health Education Specialist Competency Development

Brent Hartman, MPH, CHES
Marissa Howat, CHES
Bernie Jarriel, MA, CHES
Raffy R. Luquis, PhD, CHES
Grace Miranda, MA, CHES
Brandy Peterson, MPH, CHES
Tywanna Purkett, MA, CHES
Susie Robinson, PhD, CHES
Keiko Sakagami, EdD, CHES
Jennifer Scofield, MA, CHES
Jody Vogelzang, PhD, CHES
Cathy D. Whaley, MA, CHES

Authors and Editors of *A Competency-Based Framework for Health Education Specialists – 2010*

Chris Arthur, PhD, CHES
Donna Beal, MPH, CHES
Cam Escoffery, PhD, MPH, CHES
Patricia A. Frye, DrPH, MPA, CHES
Melissa Grim, PhD, CHES (author/editor)
Leonard Jack, Jr., PhD, MSc, CHES (author/editor)
Dennis Kamholtz, PhD, CHES
Maurice "Bud" Martin, PhD, CHES
Beverly Saxton Mahoney, RN, MS, PhD, CHES
James F. McKenzie, PhD, MPH, CHES
Angela Mickalide, PhD, CHES
Jacquie Rainey, DrPH, CHES
Rebecca Reeve, PhD, CHES
Christopher N. Thomas, MS, CHES
Tung-Sung "Sam" Tseng, DrPH, MS, CHES
Kelly Wilson, PhD, CHES
Katherine Wilson, PhD, CHES

National Health Educator Competencies Update Project (CUP): 1998-2004

CUP Steering Committee
Dr. Gary Gilmore, CUP Chair
Dr. Larry Olsen
Dr. Alyson Taub

CUP Advisory Committee
Ms. Elaine Auld
Dr. David R. Black
Dr. Tom Butler
Dr. Ellen M. Capwell
Dr. Helen Welle Graf
Ms. Barbara Hager
Ms. Linda Lysoby
Dr. Beverly Mahoney
Dr. Mary Marks
Dr. Marion Micke
Dr. Kathleen Miner
Dr. Sheila M. Patterson
Dr. Susan Radius
Dr. Edmund Ricci
Dr. John Sciacca
Dr. Becky Smith
Dr. Margaret Smith
Dr. Carol Soha
Ms. Lori Stegmier
Dr. Stephen H. Stewart
Ms. Emily Tyler

CUP Data Analysis Group
Dr. Randy Black
Dr. Dave Connell
Dr. Dan Coster
Dr. Gary Gilmore
Dr. Kathy Miner
Dr. Larry Olsen
Dr. Alyson Taub

Graduate-Level Preparation Standards Project: 1992-1998

Joint Committee for the Development of Graduate-Level Preparation Standards
Dr. Margaret M. Smith, Co-Chairperson
Dr. Stephen H. Stewart, Co-Chairperson
Dr. Evelyn E. Ames
Dr. Donald L. Calitri

Appendix C: History of Working Groups for Health Education Specialist Competency Development

Dr. William B. Cissell
Ms. Patricia P. Evans
Ms. Mary E. Hawkins
Mr. Douglas Rippler
Dr. Mark J. Kittleson
Dr. William C. Livingood, Jr.
Capt. Patricia D. Mail
Dr. Carl J. Peter
Dr. Donald A. Read
Ms. Ruth Richards
Dr. James Robinson III
Dr. Elaine M. Vitello

Graduate Competencies Writing Ad Hoc Committee
Ms. Patricia P. Evans
Dr. William C. Livingood, Jr.
Capt. Patricia D. Mail
Dr. James Robinson
Dr. Margaret M. Smith
Dr. Alyson Taub

Graduate Competencies Implementation Committee
Ms. Elaine Auld
Dr. Ellen M. Capwell
Dr. William B. Cissell
Mr. William B. Cosgrove
Ms. Patricia P. Evans
Ms. Aileen Frazee
Dr. Gary D. Gilmore
Dr. Audrey Gotsch
Dr. William C. Livingood, Jr.
Dr. Sheila M. Patterson
Dr. James Robinson
Dr. Louis Rowitz
Dr. Becky J. Smith
Dr. Margaret M. Smith
Dr. Stephen H. Stewart
Dr. Alyson Taub
Dr. Elaine M. Vitello

National Task Force on the Preparation and Practice of Health Educators: 1978-1988

Chair and Founder
Dr. Helen Cleary

Vice Chair and Co-founder
Dr. Peter Cortese

Original Task Force Members
Dr. Helen Cleary
Dr. Peter Cortese
Dr. John Burt
Dr. William Carlyon
Dr. Mabel Robinson
Dr. Helen S. Ross
Dr. Warren Schaller
Dr. Joan M. Wolle

Task Force Members
Dr. William B. Cissell
Dr. John Cooper
Dr. Bryan Cooke
Dr. Robert H. Conn
Dr. Wanda H. Jubb
Ms. Elizabeth Lee
Rev. Robert McEwen
Ms. Helen Savage
Dr. Becky J. Smith
Mr. Leonard Tritsch
Dr. Alyson Taub
Dr. Elaine M. Vitello
Ms. Anna Skiff, MPH, Volunteer Staff

Appendix C: History of Working Groups for Health Education Specialist Competency Development

Notes

Appendix D: Competency Matrices

This section contains matrices that can be used by faculty members in university programs to evaluate the degree to which their curricula address the Areas of Responsibility, Competencies, and Sub-competencies of the HESPA II 2020 Model. Completed matrices can be used by respective faculty and decision-makers to identify specific courses in which (1) the Model components are addressed and the extent to which each Competency and Sub-competency is addressed within courses and across the curriculum and (2) identified gaps in coverage can be targeted for improvement. The results can be included in accreditation reports and communicated to students in the program who are interested in understanding program strengths and learning expectations.

DIRECTIONS FOR USE OF THE AREA OF RESPONSIBILITY MATRICES

A matrix is provided in this section for each of the Eight Areas of Responsibility. Each Area of Responsibility matrix contains grids specific to the entry- and advanced-level Sub-competencies for that Area. Specific recommendations to the profession that impact curricula development can be found in Section IV of this publication. Baccalaureate degree programs should prepare graduates to perform all entry-level Competencies and Sub-competencies within the Areas of Responsibility. Master's and doctoral degree programs should prepare graduates to perform all entry- and advanced-1 level Competencies and Sub-competencies within the Areas of Responsibility. Additionally, doctoral programs should emphasize all advanced 2-level Sub-competencies. Due to the hierarchical nature of the HESPA II 2020 Model (advanced-level building on entry-level), when evaluating a program designed to prepare students for advanced-level practice, some courses will need to be listed in the entry-level grid on the matrix to indicate courses in which entry-level Sub-competencies are highlighted. Other courses will need to be listed in the advanced-level grid to indicate courses in which advanced-level Sub-competencies are emphasized. It is possible that some courses may need to be listed on both grids and that some advanced-level Sub-competencies may be addressed in a baccalaureate degree program.

To use the matrices effectively, enter the course number and title of each professional preparation course required of health education majors enrolled in your program. Only faculty members currently responsible for teaching a course should complete the matrix for that course. The designated course instructor(s) for a course should refer to the Competencies and Sub-competencies specific to each Area of Responsibility and determine whether or not each of the Sub-competencies is currently being taught as an integral part of the course. In making this determination, the course instructor(s) should note that a Competency statement does not merely represent subject matter relevant to a skill. The statement must be viewed as an actual Competency (i.e., skills and abilities). The question each instructor must answer in connection with every Competency and Sub-competency specified in the Area matrices is: "Are the students taking this course merely learning associated subject matter or are they learning to perform the described Competency (i.e., skills and abilities)?" Obviously, the instructor of each course is more qualified than any other faculty member to make that judgment. If a Sub-competency is given major emphasis as part of a course, the instructor should place the number 2 in the corresponding box. If the Sub-competency receives at least minor study and practice in the course, the number 1 should be assigned. In the event that a Sub-competency is not a part of the content of that course, a score of 0 should be assigned. The total mathematical sum of these entries for each course should be recorded in the far right column titled "Total by Course." Figure D.1 contains example entries for four health education courses.

FIGURE D.1 *Example of Area of Responsibility and Competencies Matrix Analysis*

AREA OF RESPONSIBILITY AND COMPETENCIES MATRIX (EXAMPLE)
Area I: Assessment of Needs and Capacity

ENTRY-LEVEL

Course Title	Comp 1.1 Sub-comp					Comp 1.2 Sub-comp								Comp 1.3 Sub-comp						Comp 1.4 Sub-comp				Total by Course (Max=44)*
	.1	.2	.3	.4	.5	.1	.2	.3	.4	.5	.6	.7	.8	.1	.2	.3	.4	.5	.6	.2	.3	.4	.5	
Community Health	1	2	2	2	2	2	2	1	1	1	1	1	1	2	2	2	2	2	2	2	2	2	2	36
Biostatistics	2	0	0	0	0	0	2	1	2	2	2	2	2	0	0	0	0	0	0	0	0	1	1	17
Administration of H.E.	2	2	1	1	1	1	1	0	0	0	0	0	0	2	2	2	2	2	2	2	2	2	2	28
School Health	1	1	2	1	1	1	1	1	1	1	1	1	1	2	2	2	2	2	2	2	2	2	2	33

Total by Area of Responsibility*
Should not exceed maximum (44) x number of courses

ADVANCED 1-LEVEL^

Course Title	Comp 1.2 Sub-comp .2	Comp 1.2 Sub-comp .9	Comp 1.4 Sub-comp .1	Total by Course (Max = 6)

Total by Area of Responsibility
Should not exceed maximum (6) x number of courses

Note.
2=Major Emphasis,
1=Minor Emphasis,
0=No Emphasis
*Max: Maximum number possible per course
^No Advanced 2-level Sub-competencies exist for Area of Responsibility I

Appendix D: Competency Matrices

DIRECTIONS FOR USE OF THE ANALYSIS SHEETS

When all of the Area of Responsibility matrices have been completed, the analysis sheets for entry-, advanced 1-, and advanced 2-levels should be used as an organizing and summarizing tool (see end of Appendix D). The analysis sheets are designed to facilitate organization of the combined data obtained from using the Area of Responsibility matrices. The same courses that appeared on the Area of Responsibility matrices are listed along the vertical axis. The data recorded on the matrices should be transferred to the analysis sheets and used to identify strengths and potential areas for improvement in the curriculum.

Notice that for each Area of Responsibility, the Competencies are indicated by a numbering system with the first number indicating the Area of Responsibility and the second number indicating the specific Competency within that area (for example, Competency 1.1, Competency 1.2, Competency 1.3, and Competency 1.4) across the horizontal axis. Below each Competency number is the total number of supportive Sub-competencies for that Competency. For example, in the entry-level analysis sheet, the number of Sub-competencies is 5, 7, 6 and 4 for Area of Responsibility I.)

In each completed Area of Responsibility matrix and for every course listed, enter the number of Sub-competencies given a rating of 2 and the number of those given a rating of 1 in the appropriate box (see Figure D.2). As an example, note in Figure D.1 that of five Sub-competencies specified as essential to the achievement of Competency 1.1 at the entry-level, the instructor of the Community Health course has reported that four Sub-competencies receive major emphasis (2), one Sub-competency is given at least some emphasis (1), with none identified as having no emphasis (0). On the analysis sheet (Figure D.2), the number of Sub-competencies given major emphasis (in this case, 4) is entered in the top portion of the box, and the number given minor emphasis (which is 1) is entered in the lower portion, so that it looks like a fraction (4/1).

In Fig. D1, the instructor of the Administration of Health Education course, under Competency 1.1 reported two Sub-competencies received major emphasis (2), three Sub-competencies were identified as receiving some emphasis (1). No Sub-competency was identified as having no emphasis (0). When all of the data have been entered into the analysis sheet (Figure D.2) for all of the courses, total and enter in the column at the far right of the matrix ("Course Total") the number of Sub-competencies reported as receiving major and minor emphasis with reference to each course. Note that these totals reflect the number of 2's and 1's, a frequency count, not the mathematical sum. As you total these counts, include both figures of the "fraction," so that 2/2 adds 4 to the total, whereas 2/0 would add only 2 to the total. Next, total each column vertically and enter that total number in the row labeled "Competency Total." The resulting "Course Total" represents the coverage of all Sub-competencies by course. The highest possible Course Total for each course is 114, which is the total number of entry-level Sub-competencies in the HES-PA II 2020 Model.

The "Competency Total" represents the coverage of each Sub-competency across all courses in the curriculum. This highest possible Competency Total for each Sub-competency is dependent upon the number of courses in the curricula. For example, the four Sub-competencies in Competency 1.1 multiplied by 10 courses in the curricula would generate a possible total of 40 as the Competency Total for that Sub-competency.

APPENDIX D

FIGURE D.2 *Example Analysis Sheet for Areas of Responsibility*

ANALYSIS SHEET: AREAS OF RESPONSIBILITY

ENTRY-LEVEL

Area	Area I				Area II				Area III			Area IV					Area V				Area VI						Area VII				Area VIII			Course Total.∧
Competency ➜	1.1	1.2	1.3	1.4	2.1	2.2	2.3	2.4	3.1	3.2	3.3	4.1	4.2	4.3	4.4	4.5	5.1	5.2	5.3	5.4	6.1	6.2	6.3	6.4	6.5	6.6	7.1	7.2	7.3	7.4	8.1	8.3	8.4	
# Sub-competencies	5	7	6	4	3	4	2	2	4	5	6	2	0	3	1	0	5	7	2	2	4	3	4	6	6	1	4	2	0	0	5	4	5	
Course Title ➜																																		
Community Health*	4/1	0/7	6/0	4/0																														
Biostatistics	1/0	6/1	0/0	0/2																														
Administration of H.E.	2/3	0/1	6/0	4/0																														
School Health	1/4	0/7	6/0	4/0																														
Competency Total∧∧	16	22	18	14																														
Proposed New Courses																																		

Note. ∧ Course Total: Sum of top and bottom numbers across all Sub-competencies for the course; Maximum possible course score = 114 (total number of existing Sub-competencies for Entry-level)

Top number: Number of Sub-competencies given major emphasis (number of "2s" in Area of Responsibility Matrix);

Bottom number: Number of Sub-competencies given minor emphasis (number of "1s" in Area of Responsibility Matrix)

∧∧ Competency Total: Sum of top and bottom numbers for all courses for designated competency; Maximum possible
Competency score = # of Sub-competencies x # of courses

Appendix D: Competency Matrices

PURPOSE OF THE MATRICES AND ANALYSIS SHEETS

The matrices and analysis sheets previously described can be used by decision-makers to determine the degree to which each course within a curriculum is addressing the Competencies and Sub-competencies of the Eight Areas of Responsibility. This information can be used to validate curricular strengths and identify potential ways in which the curriculum may be further developed or enhanced so that students are equipped with needed professional Competencies.

A completed analysis sheet (Figure D.2) can provide a summary of the balance of Sub-competency emphasis within each Competency of the Eight Areas of Responsibility. The top and bottom numbers in each "cell" of the analysis sheet represent that emphasis balance in each course. For example, the School Health course in Figure D.2 contains an emphasis on all five Sub-competencies in Competency 1.1; with a major emphasis on one Sub-Competency as indicated by the top number being "1" (one score of 1) and a minor emphasis on four Sub-Competencies as indicated by the bottom number being a "4" (4 scores of 1). The entry for that box is 4/1, indicating that all five Sub-competencies in Competency 1 have at least some emphasis.

The Competency Totals at the bottom of the analysis sheet can be used to identify Sub-competencies that are emphasized the most and least across the curriculum. The Course Totals in the far right column of the sheet can be used to identify the courses in which most Sub-competencies are identified. These two variables are useful in efforts to achieve a balanced approach to Sub-competency emphasis across the curriculum.

The Area of Responsibility matrices (Figure D.1) can provide more details about emphasis levels for each Sub-competency in each course. This information can be useful in determining whether emphasis levels are appropriate in specific courses. If, for example, the Community Health course was previously designated by decision-makers as the course within the curriculum where most emphasis on assessment concepts should be made, a lesser number of zeros (0) or ones (1) in the row for that course within the Area I (Assessment of needs and capacity) matrix could warrant a need for discussion about whether more emphasis for those Sub-competencies in that course is needed. The matrix also can be used to quickly note emphasis levels across courses for a Sub-competency, with the discovery of a large number of zeros or ones in a specific Sub-competency column possibly warranting discussion.

ADAPTING EXISTING CURRICULA

The Curriculum Decision-Making Matrix in Figure D.3 contains a list of questions faculty members may use to summarize findings and determine any necessary actions. It is possible that existing courses in a traditional professional preparation program in health education would not have to be significantly changed to adopt a Competency-based plan. Rather, a need for a new perspective on course goals and objectives and increased use of experiential teaching-learning methods to address the Competency-based Model would be more likely. All of the Competencies for each Area of Responsibility should be included in some instructional activity in a course.

The whole faculty should engage in curriculum design and analysis to enhance consistency in how the Sub-competencies are addressed across the curriculum. Each faculty member responsible for a course should be charged with making any revisions needed to better the fit between course objectives and designated Sub-competencies. All faculty members should participate in planning and designing any new courses deemed necessary to emphasize Sub-competencies currently overlooked. Though Knowledge items are not currently used in curriculum analyses, the verified Knowledge items in Section VI of this document may be useful in course development.

Appendix D: Competency Matrices

FIGURE D.3 *Sample Questions for Curriculum Decision-Making*

	CURRICULUM DECISION-MAKING MATRIX		
#	Question	Findings	Needed Action
1	How many of the Competencies are currently being addressed by the curriculum?		
2	How many of the Sub-competencies receive major emphasis in the program, as shown by a rating of 2?		
3	How many of the Sub-competencies receive at least minor study, as shown by a rating of 1?		
4	If there are Competencies not currently receiving any attention at all, which are they, and in what Area(s) are they found?		
5	In each of the Areas of Responsibility, how many Sub-Competencies are not being addressed?		
6	Which courses are providing broadest coverage and which are providing least coverage of the Eight Areas of Responsibility?		
7	Are there any Areas of Responsibility that now receive little if any consideration in the curriculum? If so, which ones?		
8	Are there courses that appear to be irrelevant to the Competencies, as reflected in the number of zeros shown? If so, could this be changed without giving up the course itself?		
9	What implications do you see in these data for course revision, course modification, or the development of a new course?		

Appendix D: Competency Matrices

DEVELOPING NEW CURRICULA

Individuals charged with developing a new curriculum for health education specialists that did not previously exist should begin with a professional preparation curriculum recommended by national health education leaders or by examining curricula of accredited programs. A careful examination of the Sub-competencies across all Eight Areas of Responsibility and discussions with national leaders in program accreditation is recommended prior to curriculum development. The verified Knowledge items described in Section VI will be useful in this effort.

In arriving at decisions about where a Competency is to be taught, it is advisable to take an experimental approach. That is, decisions reached at this point need to be regarded as tentative and subject to change through trial and evaluation by students, faculty members, alumni, advisory groups, and employers of program graduates. Several years of evaluation and modification may be necessary before there is assurance that the curriculum is providing opportunities for optimal Competency development. The faculty members also should note that the Competency-based Framework for Health Education Specialists is updated through national studies on a regular basis to ensure that the Competency Model used to frame curricula accurately reflects professional practice.

SELECTING TEACHING-LEARNING STRATEGIES

It is not the function of a curriculum framework to specify or describe learning opportunities or lesson plans. But rather, a curriculum framework outlines what should be taught—not how to teach it. It is the responsibility of those who deliver the curriculum to select the strategies to be used. Criteria for the selection of a teaching strategy include the following: (a) it must provide practice in the skill specified in the objective; (b) it must arrange for the discovery or introduction of the content; (c) the activities must be satisfying to the learner; and (d) the activities must be appropriate to the past experiences and present abilities of the learner. If several strategies meet the preceding criteria, the one chosen should be the strategy most likely to produce more than one positive outcome. In general, experiential learning is more effective than passive learning in promoting competency. That is, most people learn better by doing than by watching or listening. The best teaching-learning strategy is the one that provides the learners with a sound understanding of the concept being taught and encourages learners to practice doing what the objective proposes that they need to be competent.

THE COMPETENCY-BASED FRAMEWORK BY AREAS OF RESPONSIBILITY

Each of the Eight Areas of Responsibility constituting the Competency-based curriculum framework is introduced by a discussion of each Area in Section III. In that section, a general statement is provided that describes each of the Areas of Responsibility in terms of its purpose, meaning, application in health education practice, and relation to the other Areas. The Competency framework for each Area is developed hierarchically as a set of Competency statements, each of which is supported by more specific and narrowly drawn Sub-competencies, upon which measurable general objectives are based and proposed. The sequence in which the Areas of Responsibility is presented is more or less logical, but not absolute. No priorities are intended, nor should any be presumed.

FIGURE D.4 Area of Responsibility I Matrix

AREA OF RESPONSIBILITY AND COMPETENCIES MATRIX
Area I: Assessment of Needs and Capacity

ENTRY-LEVEL

Course Title	Comp 1.1 Sub-comp					Comp 1.2 Sub-comp									Comp 1.3 Sub-comp						Comp 1.4 Sub-comp				Total by Course (Max=44)*
	.1	.2	.3	.4	.5	.1	.2	.3	.4	.5	.6	.7	.8	.1	.2	.3	.4	.5	.6	.1	.2	.3	.4	.5	
Community Health																									
Biostatistics																									
Administration of H.E.																									
School Health																									
Total by Area of Responsibility*																									

Should not exceed maximum (44) x number of courses

ADVANCED 1-LEVEL^

Course Title	Comp 1.2 Sub-comp .2	Sub-comp .9	Comp 1.4 Sub-comp .1	Total by Course (Max = 6)
Total by Area of Responsibility				

Should not exceed maximum (6) x number of courses

Note.
2=Major Emphasis,
1=Minor Emphasis,
0=No Emphasis
*Max: Maximum number possible per course
^No Advanced 2-level Sub-competencies exist for Area of Responsibility I

Appendix D: Competency Matrices

FIGURE D.5 *Area of Responsibility II Matrix*

AREA OF RESPONSIBILITY AND COMPETENCIES MATRIX
Area II: Planning

ENTRY-LEVEL

Course Title	Comp 2.1 Sub-comp			Comp 2.2 Sub-comp				Comp 2.3 Sub-comp		Comp 2.4 Sub-comp		Total by Course (Max=22)*
	.1	.2	.3	.1	.2	.3	.4	.1	.4	.2	.3	
Total by Area of Responsibility*												
Should not exceed maximum (22) x number of courses												

ADVANCED 1-LEVEL^

Course Title	Comp 2.3 Sub-comp				Comp 2.4 Sub-comp			Total by Course (Max=16)
	.2	.3	.5	.6	.7	.1	.4	.5
Total by Area of Responsibility								
Should not exceed maximum (16) x number of courses								

Note.
2=Major Emphasis,
1=Minor Emphasis,
0=No Emphasis
*Max: Maximum number possible per course
^No Advanced 2-level Sub-competencies exist for Area of Responsibility II

APPENDIX D

FIGURE D.6 *Area of Responsibility III Matrix*

AREA OF RESPONSIBILITY AND COMPETENCIES MATRIX
Area III: Implementation

ENTRY-LEVEL

Course Title	Comp 3.1					Comp 3.2					Comp 3.3						Total by Course (Max=30)
	Sub-comp					Sub-comp					Sub-comp						
	.1	.2	.3		.5	.1	.2	.3	.4	.5	.1	.2	.3	.4	.5	.6	
Total by Area of Responsibility																	

Should not exceed maximum (30) x number of courses

ADVANCED 1-LEVEL^

Course Title	Comp 3.1	Total by Course (Max = 2)
	Sub-comp .4	
Total by Area of Responsibility		

Should not exceed maximum (2) x number of courses

Note.
2=Major Emphasis,
1=Minor Emphasis,
0=No Emphasis
*Max: Maximum number possible per course
^No Advanced 2-level Sub-competencies exist for Area of Responsibility III

FIGURE D.7a Area of Responsibility IV Matrix

AREA OF RESPONSIBILITY AND COMPETENCIES MATRIX
Area IV: Evaluation and Research

ENTRY-LEVEL

Note.
2=Major Emphasis,
1=Minor Emphasis,
0=No Emphasis
*Max: Maximum number possible per course

Course Title	Comp 4.1 Sub-comp					Comp 4.3 Sub-comp			Comp 4.4 Sub-comp	Total by Course (Max=12)
	.2	.8	.4	.3		.2	.3	.5	.3	

Total by Area of Responsibility
Should not exceed maximum (12) x number of courses

AREA IV: ADVANCED 1-LEVEL

Course Title	Comp 4.1 Sub-comp							Comp 4.2 Sub-comp						Comp 4.4 Sub-comp	Comp 4.5 Sub-comp	Total by Course (Max=32)*
	.1	.3	.4	.5	.6	.7	.9	.10	.2	.3	.5	.6	.7	.2	.1	.4

Total by Area of Responsibility
Should not exceed maximum (32) x number of courses

FIGURE D.7b *Area of Responsibility IV: Advanced 2-Level Matrix*

AREA OF RESPONSIBILITY AND COMPETENCIES MATRIX
Area IV: Evaluation and Research

AREA IV: ADVANCED 2-LEVEL

Course Title	Comp 4.2 Sub-comp			Comp 4.3 Sub-comp				Comp 4.4 Sub-comp						Comp 4.5 Sub-comp		Total by Course (Max=30)
	.1	.4	.8	.9	.1	.4	.6	.1	.4	.5	.6	.7	.8	.2	.3	

Total by Area of Responsibility
Should not exceed maximum (30) x number of courses

Note.
2=Major Emphasis,
1=Minor Emphasis,
0=No Emphasis
*Max: Maximum number possible per course

FIGURE D.8 *Area of Responsibility V Matrix*

AREA OF RESPONSIBILITY AND COMPETENCIES MATRIX
Area V: Advocacy

ENTRY-LEVEL

Course Title	Comp 5.1 Sub-comp					Comp 5.2 Sub-comp								Comp 5.3 Sub-comp		Comp 5.4 Sub-comp		Total by Course (Max=32)*
	.1	.2	.3	.4	.5	.1	.2	.4	.5	.6	.7	.8		.1	.2	.1	.2	
Total by Area of Responsibility *Should not exceed maximum (32) x number of courses*																		

ADVANCED 1-LEVEL^

Course Title	Comp 5.2 Sub-comp .3	Comp 5.3 Sub-comp .3	Total by Course (Max = 4)*
Total by Area of Responsibility *Should not exceed maximum (4) x number of courses*			

Note.
2=Major Emphasis,
1=Minor Emphasis,
0=No Emphasis
*Max: Maximum number possible per course
^No Advanced 2-level Sub-competencies exist for Area of Responsibility V

FIGURE D.9 Area of Responsibility VI Matrix

AREA OF RESPONSIBILITY AND COMPETENCIES MATRIX
Area VI: Communication

ENTRY-LEVEL

Course Title	Comp 6.1 Sub-comp				Comp 6.2 Sub-comp			Comp 6.3 Sub-comp				Comp 6.4 Sub-comp						Comp 6.5						Comp 6.6	Total by Course (Max=48)*
	.1	.2	.3	.4	.1	.2	.3	.1	.2	.3	.4	.1	.2	.3	.4	.5	.6	.1	.2	.3	.4	.5	.6	.1	

Total by Area of Responsibility
Should not exceed maximum (48) x number of courses

ADVANCED 1-LEVEL | ADVANCED 2-LEVEL

Course Title	Comp 6.6 Sub-comp .3	Comp 6.6 Sub-comp .2	Total by Course (Max = 4)*

Total by Area of Responsibility
Should not exceed maximum (4) x number of courses

Note.
2=Major Emphasis,
1=Minor Emphasis,
0=No Emphasis
*Max: Maximum number possible per course

FIGURE D.10 *Area of Responsibility VII Matrix*

AREA OF RESPONSIBILITY AND COMPETENCIES MATRIX
Area VII: Leadership and Management

Note.
2=Major Emphasis,
1=Minor Emphasis,
0=No Emphasis
*Max: Maximum number possible per course

ENTRY-LEVEL

Course Title	Comp 7.1 Sub-comp					Comp 7.2 Sub-comp		Total by Course (Max=12)*
	.1	.2	.3	.5		.1	.2	

Total by Area of Responsibility
Should not exceed maximum (12) x number of courses

ADVANCED 1-LEVEL

Course Title	Comp 7.1 Sub-comp	Comp 7.2 Sub-comp			Comp 7.3 Sub-comp								Comp 7.4 Sub-comp								
	.4	.3	.4	.5	6	.1	.2	.3	.4	.5	.6	.7	.1	.2	.3	.5	.7	.8	.9		

ADVANCED 2-LEVEL

	Comp 7.5 Sub-comp			Comp 7.4 Sub-comp		Total by Course (Max = 50)*
	.1	.2	.3	.4	.6	

Total by Area of Responsibility
Should not exceed maximum (50) x number of courses

FIGURE D.11 *Area of Responsibility VIII Matrix*

AREA OF RESPONSIBILITY AND COMPETENCIES MATRIX
Area VIII: Ethics and Professionalism

ENTRY-LEVEL

Course Title	Comp 8.1				Comp 8.3				Comp 8.4				Total by Course (Max=28)
	Sub-comp				Sub-comp				Sub-comp				
	.3	.4	.5	.6	.1	.2	.3	.4	.1	.2	.3	.4	.5	

Total by Area of Responsibility
Should not exceed maximum (28) x number of courses

ADVANCED 1-LEVEL / **ADVANCED 2-LEVEL**

Course Title	Comp 8.1	Comp 8.2	Comp 8.4	Comp 8.2	Comp 8.3	Total by Course (Max = 14)*
	Sub-comp	Sub-comp	Sub-comp	Sub-comp	Sub-comp	
	.2	.1	.2	.6	.7	.3	.5	

Total by Area of Responsibility
Should not exceed maximum (14) x number of courses

Note.
2=Major Emphasis,
1=Minor Emphasis,
0=No Emphasis
*Max: Maximum number possible per course

Appendix D: Competency Matrices

FIGURE D.12 *Analysis Sheet: Area of Responsibility, Entry-Level*

ANALYSIS SHEET: AREAS OF RESPONSIBILITY

ENTRY-LEVEL

Area	Area I				Area II				Area III			Area IV					Area V				Area VI						Area VII				Area VIII			Course Total^
Competency →	1.1	1.2	1.3	1.4	2.1	2.2	2.3	2.4	3.1	3.2	3.3	4.1	4.2	4.3	4.4	4.5	5.1	5.2	5.3	5.4	6.1	6.2	6.3	6.4	6.5	6.6	7.1	7.2	7.3	7.4	8.1	8.3	8.4	
# Sub-competencies	5	7	6	4	3	4	2	2	4	5	6	2	0	3	1	0	5	7	2	2	4	3	4	6	6	1	4	2	0	0	5	4	5	
Course Title →																																		
Competency Total^^ →																																		
Proposed New Courses																																		

Note. Top number: Number of Sub-competencies given major emphasis (number of "2s" in Area of Responsibility Matrix);
Bottom number: Number of Sub-competencies given minor emphasis (number of "1s" in Area of Responsibility Matrix)
^ Course Total: Sum of top and bottom numbers across all Sub-competencies for the course; Maximum possible course score = 114 (total number of existing Sub-competencies for Entry-level)
^^ Competency Total: Sum of top and bottom numbers for all courses for designated Competency; Maximum possible competency score = # of Sub-competencies x # of courses

FIGURE D.13 *Analysis Sheet: Areas of Responsibility, Advanced 1-level*

ANALYSIS SHEET: AREAS OF RESPONSIBILITY

ADVANCED 1-LEVEL

Area	Area I				Area II				Area III			Area IV					Area V				Area VI						Area VII					Area VIII			Course Total∧
Competency →	1.1	1.2	1.3	1.4	2.1	2.2	2.3	2.4	3.1	3.2	3.3	4.1	4.2	4.3	4.4	4.5	5.1	5.2	5.3	5.4	6.1	6.2	6.3	6.4	6.5	6.6	7.1	7.2	7.3	7.4	7.5	8.1	8.3	8.4	
# Sub-competencies	0	2	0	1	0	0	5	3	1	0	0	8	5	0	1	2	0	1	1	0	0	0	0	0	0	1	1	4	8	7	3	1	2	2	2
Course Title																																			
Community Health *																																			
Biostatistics																																			
Administration of H.E.																																			
School Health																																			
Competency Total∧∧																																			
Proposed New Courses																																			

Note. Top number: Number of Sub-competencies given <u>major</u> emphasis (number of "2s" in Area of Responsibility Matrix);
Bottom number: Number of Sub-competencies given <u>minor</u> emphasis (number of "1s" in Area of Responsibility Matrix
∧ Course Total: Sum of top and bottom numbers across all Sub-competencies for the course; Maximum possible course score = 59 (total number of existing Sub-competencies for Advanced 1-level)
∧∧ Competency Total: Sum of top and bottom numbers for all courses for designated Competency; Maximum possible competency score = # of Sub-competencies x # of courses

Appendix D: Competency Matrices

FIGURE D.14 *Analysis Sheet: Areas of Responsibility, Advanced 2-level*

ANALYSIS SHEET: AREAS OF RESPONSIBILITY
ADVANCED 2-LEVEL

Area	Area I				Area II				Area III			Area IV					Area V				Area VI						Area VII					Area VIII				Course Total^
Competency →	1.1	1.2	1.3	1.4	2.1	2.2	2.3	2.4	3.1	3.2	3.3	4.1	4.2	4.3	4.4	4.5	5.1	5.2	5.3	5.4	6.1	6.2	6.3	6.4	6.5	6.6	7.1	7.2	7.3	7.4	7.5	8.1	8.2	8.3	8.4	
# Sub-competencies	0	0	0	0	0	0	0	0	0	0	0	0	4	3	6	2	0	0	0	0	0	0	0	0	0	1	0	0	0	2	0	0	1	1	0	0
Course Title →																																				
Community* Health																																				
Biostatistics																																				
Administration of H.E.																																				
School Health																																				
Competency Total^^ →																																				
Proposed New Courses																																				

Note. * Areas of Responsibility I, II, III, V, and VI do not contain Advanced 2-level Sub-competencies

••Top number: Number of Sub-competencies given major emphasis (number of "2s" in Area of Responsibility Matrix)

Bottom number: Number of Sub-competencies given minor emphasis (number of "1s" in Area of Responsibility Matrix)

^ Course Total: Sum of top and bottom numbers across all Sub-competencies for the course; Maximum possible course score = 20 (total number of existing Sub-competencies for Advanced 2-level)

^^ Competency Total: Sum of top and bottom numbers for all courses for designated Competency; Maximum possible Competency score = # of Sub-competencies x # of courses

APPENDIX D

Appendix D: Competency Matrices

APPENDIX D

Notes